Group Play Therapy

Group Play Therapy presents an updated look at an effective yet underutilized therapeutic intervention. More than just an approach to treating children, group play therapy is a life-span approach, undergirded by solid theory and, in this volume, taking wings through exciting techniques. Drawing on their experiences as clinicians and educators, the authors weave theory and technique together to create a valuable resource for both mental health practitioners and advanced students. Therapists and ultimately their clients will benefit from enhancing their understanding of group play therapy.

Daniel S. Sweeney, PhD, is a professor of counseling and director of the Northwest Center for Play Therapy Studies at George Fox University in Portland, Oregon. He is a past board member and president of the Association for Play Therapy. Dr. Sweeney maintains a small private practice and is an international presenter. He has authored or co-authored several books, including *Play Therapy Interventions with Children's Problems, Counseling Children Through the World of Play, Sandtray Therapy: A Practical Manual,* and *The Handbook of Group Play Therapy.* His books have been translated into Chinese, Korean, and Russian.

Jennifer N. Baggerly, PhD, is a professor and the chair of the division of counseling and human services at the University of North Texas at Dallas and has served as chair of the board of directors of the Association for Play Therapy. She has taught and provided group play therapy for over ten years in schools and community agencies. Dr. Baggerly's multiple research projects and over fifty publications have led to her being recognized as a prominent play therapy expert.

Dee C. Ray, PhD, is a professor in the counseling program and director of the Child and Family Resource Clinic at the University of North Texas. Dr. Ray has published over seventy-five articles, chapters, and books in the field of play therapy, and over twenty research publications specifically examining the effects of child-centered play therapy. Dr. Ray is the author of *Advanced Play Therapy,* co-editor of *Child Centered Play Therapy Research,* and former editor of the *International Journal of Play Therapy.*

Group Play Therapy

A Dynamic Approach

Daniel S. Sweeney,
Jennifer N. Baggerly, and Dee C. Ray

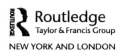

Routledge
Taylor & Francis Group

NEW YORK AND LONDON

First published 2014
by Routledge
711 Third Avenue, New York, NY 10017

and by Routledge
27 Church Road, Hove, East Sussex BN3 2FA

Library of Congress Cataloging in Publication Data
Sweeney, Daniel S.
  Group play therapy : a dynamic approach / Daniel S. Sweeney, Jennifer N. Baggerly, and
  Dee C. Ray.
    pages cm
  Includes bibliographical references and index.
  1. Group play therapy. I. Baggerly, Jennifer. II. Ray, Dee C. III. Title.
  RJ505.P6S94 2014
  618.92'891653—dc23
  2013022601

ISBN: 978-0-415-62481-7 (hbk)
ISBN: 978-0-415-65785-3 (pbk)
ISBN: 978-0-203-10394-4 (ebk)

Typeset in Minion
by EvS Communication Networx, Inc.

For Garry Landreth, a common mentor and friend to the three of us, who has both taught and modeled relationship. We walk different paths, but follow a similar vision and mission—to help make the world a little safer for children.

Contents

Foreword

In 1999, I wrote "Although the field of play therapy has made great strides since the ground-breaking work of pioneers in the early 1900s, little has been done to facilitate the development of group play therapy. There has been to my knowledge only one group play therapy text published in the past seventy-five years" (Landreth, 1999, p. xi). Although Sweeney and Homeyer (1999) published an edited group play therapy text that year, the statement is still largely true. The dearth of emphasis and publications on group play therapy continues to puzzle me.

Just as play is the natural medium of expression for children in therapy, a group, defined in play therapy as two or more children, is the natural medium for building a relationship for many children in need of therapy. Our society, indeed any society, is built on relationships and is only as strong as those relationships. Military forces, gigantic corporations, and powerful political groups are not the life blood of a society. Relationships that exist in a family group are the dynamic energy that propels a society forward. In like manner, a play therapy group facilitates the creative expression of children's "innate inner-directional, constructive, forward moving, creative, self-healing movement toward growth" (Landreth, 2012, p. 54).

Group play therapy provides unique possibilities and therapeutic advantages not available in typical individual play therapy experiences. Some cautious, abused, or traumatized children do not feel safe alone with a play therapist, and even the warmest, most caring, and experienced play therapist may not be given an opportunity to enter the child's world and make contact with the inner emotional person of the child that lies hidden behind a rigid defense mechanism that protects the child. Such children often feel more quickly safe with a peer and are drawn into the other child's or other children's activities in the playroom. The result is dynamic expression and exploration.

Individuals function most of their lives within some sort of group. Against this background of interaction with others, the child's self-concept is formed and many times distorted. This distorted perception of self, and self in relation to others, often occurs in the dynamics of the family group relationship. Therefore, since perception is the basis for behavior and perceptions are changed as a result of meaningful relationships, the most effective place for dealing with behavioral issues may be within a relationship that incorporates the basic structure which originally contributed to the difficulty. The power of interpersonal relationships to change perception is graphically described in *The Little Prince* (de Saint Exupery, 1943). In the story, the fox tells the little prince about his life and says,

But if you tame me [build a relationship with me: my interpretation], it will be as if the sun came to shine on my life. I shall know the sound of a step that will be different from all the others. Other steps send me hurrying back underneath the ground. Yours will call me, like music, out of my burrow. And then look: you see the grain-fields down yonder? I do not eat bread. Wheat is of no use to me. The wheat fields have nothing to say to me. And that is sad. But you have hair that is the color of gold. Think how wonderful that will be when you have tamed me! The grain, which is also golden, will bring me back the thought of you. And I shall love to listen to the wind in the wheat.

(p. 83)

This is a wonderful description of what occurs in the process of group play therapy. Sweeney, Baggerly, and Ray have interwoven this concept into the fabric of the chapters of this book. Their writings in these chapters highlight group play therapy as an extraordinary process for facilitating the growth of children and in the process of accomplishing this task they provide an integration of theory and practice in group play therapy. This is the only book in published literature that describes various theoretical approaches or adaptations to group play therapy and shows how each would respond to or deal with the same problematic happenings in a group play therapy situation. This practical book is a must-read resource for elementary school counselors, psychologists, social workers, counselors, and other mental health professionals who work with children.

In the pages of this book, we are privileged to experience child and therapist interactions that clearly demonstrate the impact of children on each other and therapists' responses to children's difficult behaviors. Topics and issues in group play therapy come alive in the interactions of Melissa, Allison, Miguel, and other children. Do you want to know how to respond to complex happenings in group play therapy? Just listen to what the children in this book say or do and how a sensitive, caring play therapist responds. If you stop to listen, you will be taught by the creative ability of Sweeney, Baggerly, and Ray to enter fully into the private world of children.

Group Play Therapy: A Dynamic Approach is THE definitive text on group play therapy. You will find the answers to your questions about group play therapy in the pages of this book.

Garry L. Landreth
Regents Professor Emeritus
University of North Texas

Preface

Psychologist and philosopher William James (1891) posits the following painful scenario:

> No more fiendish punishment could be devised, were such a thing physically possible, than that one should be turned loose in society and remain absolutely unnoticed by all the members thereof. If no one turned round when we entered, answered when we spoke, or minded what we did, but if every person we met 'cut us dead,' and acted as if we were non-existing things, a kind of rage and impotent despair would ere long well up in us, from which the cruelest bodily tortures would be a relief.
>
> (pp. 293–294)

One of the greatest places of pain for all humanity is the loneliness of being alone, to feel "absolutely unnoticed". All therapists—perhaps more so, play therapists—have the responsibility, the privilege, and the honor of touching this place of loneliness in the hearts of clients. Particularly child clients, who are the common recipients of play therapy. Group therapists—perhaps more so, group play therapists—have great potential to touch the lives of those oppressed by the cruelty of isolation and loneliness, so often caused by community and paradoxically healed by community.

It is challenging to talk about group therapy without beginning with these comments about loneliness and aloneness. In his discussion of loneliness, Clark Moustakas (1974) poignantly stated: "It is the terror of loneliness, not loneliness itself but loneliness anxiety, the fear of being left alone, of being left out, that represents a dominant crisis in the struggle to become a person" (p. 16). Sweeney (2011a) suggests:

> While group play therapy cannot be classified as a specific technique or as a particular theoretical approach, it does create the opportunity for the loneliness of struggle to be addressed in a developmentally appropriate and expressive manner. Group play therapy is the recognition of children's medium of communication (play), combined with the natural benefit of human connection with other children, under the facilitation of a trained and caring adult.
>
> (p. 227)

Group play therapy is not new. When Samuel Slavson (1948) was conducting and writing about group play therapy in the 1940s, he said that the "specific advantage of the group in play therapy lies in the catalytic effect that each patient has upon the other" (p. 320)—touching that place of loneliness that both children and adults struggle with. Slavson goes on to say that play therapy group members "assign themselves to roles which are reflections or extensions of their basic problems … and find easy and natural means of coming through in a variety of play forms and activity channels" (p. 320).

Slavson's assertions are echoed by Haim Ginott, who wrote the first book on group play therapy, *Group Psychotherapy with Children: The Theory and Practice of Play Therapy* (1961). In an earlier article, Ginott (1958) wrote: "in play group therapy the presence of other children seems to relax the atmosphere, diminish the tension, and stimulate activity and participation" (p. 411). This promotes relationship, which is not only a common thread throughout this book, but the foundation of all psychotherapy, whether individual or group.

While this book primarily focuses on group play therapy with children, it is important to note that play therapy interventions can be used with all ages. It is also essential to note that group play therapy is not tied to a particular theoretical orientation or therapeutic approach. This does not make group play therapy atheoretical but rather cross-theoretical. It is not tied to a narrow set of therapeutic interventions or technical applications, but rather has incredible potential for adaptation and utilization. This book will explore many, but certainly not all possible group play therapy interventions.

This points to principles we believe are crucial in regard to therapeutic techniques. Sweeney (2011a) emphasizes that theory is always important, but theory without technique is basically philosophy. At the same time techniques may be quite valuable, but techniques without theory are reckless, and could be damaging. Sweeney goes on to suggest:

> Group play therapists as well as all therapists are encouraged to ponder some questions regarding employing techniques: (a) Is the technique developmentally appropriate? [which presupposes that developmental capabilities are a key therapeutic consideration]; (b) What theory underlies the technique? [which presupposes that techniques should be theory-based]; and (c) What is the therapeutic intent in employing a given technique? [which presupposes that having specific therapeutic intent is clinically and ethically important].
>
> (p.236)

Thus, as we talk about both directive and nondirective interventions, we strongly encourage group play therapists ask themselves these important questions. We don't have to necessarily agree on the answers to these questions, but asking and answering them makes for clinically and ethically sound therapeutic decisions.

We would suggest that group therapy, despite its long history and significant value is considerably underutilized. It is our hope that this book will not only assist readers in terms of understanding and skill development, but also serve as inspiration to use group play therapy with children, adolescents, and adults. We challenge ourselves— and you—to continue your hard work with clients, and include group play therapy as part of your therapeutic milieu.

Acknowledgments

As we explore the power of working with groups, I would like to acknowledge and thank the primary groups in my life. First, the group I love so dearly, my family—my beautiful wife Marla, and my incredible children—Jessica and Ryan, Michele and Adam, Renata, and Josiah. Second, I am so grateful for my colleagues and students in the Graduate Department of Counseling at George Fox University. And finally, I must thank my spiritual and faith community at New Vision Fellowship and the Oregon Free Methodist Conference. My family, friends, and faith are what make professional endeavors possible.

Daniel Sweeney

A group or pod of dolphins takes turns protecting and propelling each other for survival and playful purpose. I acknowledge and thank my original pod members of my mother Jean Louise Baggerly, my father Leo Baggerly, and my brother Philip M. Baggerly, as well as my current pod members of my daughter Katelyn Jean Baggerly and my partner Beth A. Kelly. I also thank my professional pod of colleagues with the University of North Texas at Dallas and the Association for Play Therapy. Thank you all for helping me surface for air, leap out of the water, and spin in the sun!

Jennifer Baggerly

Relationship is the foundation of group. It is within relationships that we see ourselves, nurture each other, and grow to our potential. I am fortunate to be in relationships that are essential to my being and inspire my work. I would like to thank the students and faculty at the University of North Texas who allow me to experience the power of group every day. I thank those in my family who nurture my soul and being—my husband Russ, and my sons, Elijah and Noah. It is my sincere hope that this book will encourage play therapists to build nurturing and attuned relationships with the groups of children we serve.

Dee Ray

1 Introduction to Group Play Therapy

Group play therapy is a cross-theoretical play therapy intervention that can and should be used by trained therapists. It encompasses a wide variety of approaches and orientations, and allows for both theoretical and technical eclecticism with a range of clients from across the developmental scale. This book will consider many dimensions of group play therapy, but is still a foundation upon which to base a considerable variety of interventions.

Sweeney and Homeyer (1999) advocate for group play therapy in their edited book, *The Handbook of Group Play Therapy*:

> Group play therapy is a natural union of two effective therapeutic modalities. Play therapists and group therapists share several important traits. Both are committed to a therapeutic process that is creative and dynamic. Both are centered on the development and maintenance of safe and therapeutic relationships. Both are focused on facilitation of an unfolding process, as opposed to the application of an immediate solution. Both are engaged in efforts requiring prerequisite training and supervision. The marriage of play therapy and group process is a natural and intuitive response to the needs of emotionally hurting children.
>
> (p. 3)

Arguably, the partnership Sweeney and Homeyer suggest is too rarely exercised. We would contend that group play therapy is not only a powerful therapeutic intervention, but it often provides a more compelling and expedient milieu than individual therapy—with both children and adults.

Group play therapy deals not only with presenting problems, but also with conscious and unconscious motivations, with the goal of insight, behavior shifts, and personality change. Groups can be focused around themes, diagnostic areas, skills development, reduction of negative emotions or behaviors, or a variety of issues. Having said this, however, we are firmly committed to a perspective that is growth-oriented, and one that is person-focused as opposed to problem-focused. While it can be argued that this is a theoretical perspective, we believe that this focus should be cross-theoretical. Fundamentally, when any therapeutic process focuses on a problem or diagnosis, the causes of the problem, or the symptomatic results of the problem, the client and the development of relationship with the client is at least minimized, and possibly lost.

This is more than sentiment; rather, it is the core of therapy. While this book will focus in many places on academic material and clinical technique, it is important that we emphasize this focus.

Group play therapy is more than an approach to working with children, adolescents, and adults. It is a process of exploration that group members embark upon, and the therapist has the privilege of partnering in. While the therapist may direct the group play therapy process, the underlying premise is that the therapist is a witness to the process, a fellow sojourner with the group members. It is upon this attitude that group members feel safe to explore, both with the therapist and with other group members. Sweeney and Landreth (2005) suggest that play therapy: "is not a cloak the play therapist puts on when entering the playroom and takes off when leaving; rather it is a philosophy resulting in attitudes and behaviors for living one's life in relationships with children" (p. 123). So it is with group play therapy and therapists, with clients of all ages.

Definition of Group Play Therapy

Defining group play therapy needs to begin with a definition of play therapy. There are several definitions for play therapy, but we have chosen Landreth's (2012) definition. Although Landreth comes from a specific theoretical orientation, his definition is arguably cross-theoretical and offers a solid basis for a definition of group play therapy. Landreth's definition is:

> Play therapy is defined as a dynamic interpersonal relationship between a child (or person of any age) and a therapist trained in play therapy procedures who provides selected play materials and facilitates the development of a safe relationship for the child (or person of any age) to fully express and explore self (feelings, thoughts, experiences, and behaviors) through play, the child's natural medium of communication, for optimal growth and development.
>
> (p. 11)

Sweeney (1997, 2011a) expands upon this definition. We firmly believe that all therapy should be *dynamic and interpersonal*. Relationship is arguably the most curative element in psychotherapy, and indeed should be an element of all approaches. In group play therapy, there is the inherent benefit to a multitude of relationships, in addition to the therapist–client relationship.

The play therapist must be *trained in play therapy procedures*. While this should be an obvious factor, it is unfortunately often overlooked. All too often, therapists using projective and expressive techniques such as play therapy have too little training, and often an embarrassing paucity of supervised experience. The group play therapist obviously needs to be trained in both play therapy and group therapy. One of these is wholly inadequate.

Play therapists must *provide selected play materials*. It is insufficient to provide a random collection of toys. Landreth (2012) reminds us that toys should be selected, not collected. Group play therapy materials should be intentionally gathered, consistent with the theoretical rationale and specific therapeutic intent. Just as the general therapy process, expressive media should be congruous with therapeutic goals and objectives.

Therapy of any kind should *facilitate the development of a safe relationship* with clients. Clients who are in a state of transition, experiencing chaos, or navigating the challenge of trauma need a place of safety because people do not grow where they do not feel safe. Facilitation brings about this place of safety. This is true for both directive and nondirective therapeutic interventions.

Within this context of safety, clients can *fully express and explore self,* which is the basis for further therapeutic advancement. We would argue that if insight and behavioral change are therapeutic goals, the ability to express and explore self is foundational. In group play therapy, of course, clients not only get to explore and express self, they get to explore others, be explored by others, express self to others, and experience other's expression of self.

Play is indeed a *child's natural medium of communication.* This is a key element of play therapy. It is also, however, a key means of communication for clients who have a challenging time verbalizing for a variety of reasons. This is what makes expressive and projective interventions so exciting for clients of all ages. In group play therapy, this dynamic is magnified, which will be further discussed below.

These elements collectively create an environment that stimulates *optimal growth and development.* This again is a cross-theoretical goal of therapy, for clients of all ages.

Sweeney (2011a) uses Landreth's (2012) definition as the basis for a group play therapy definition. For the purposes of this book, group play therapy is defined as:

> A dynamic, interpersonal, and reciprocal relationship between two or more clients and a therapist trained in both play therapy and group therapy procedures. This involves the selection of specific expressive and projective play media, and the facilitation and development of safe relationships for clients to express and explore themselves and others (including feelings, thoughts, experiences, and behaviors). This occurs through expressive play, a natural medium of communication for children and a nonverbal means of expression for persons of all ages.

Rationale for Play Therapy

Without knowing the background of this book's readers, it seems important to summarize the basic rationale for play therapy, before explaining the rationale for group play therapy. Sweeney (1997) and Homeyer and Sweeney (2011) list several.

1. Play is the child's natural medium of communication. This is opposed to "adult therapy," which presupposes the client's ability to engage verbally and cognitively, and process abstract concepts. Children are developmentally different than adults, and do not communicate the same way adults do. To expect children to leave their world of play and enter the adult world of communication is fundamentally dishonoring.
2. This is also true for the verbally precocious child as well. It is an error to assume that children who appear to have verbal skills are therefore able to express their

emotional lives in words. Their verbal abilities may be a reflection of advanced intelligence or parentification (or a variety of other sources). This does not mean that words are the appropriate means of relational connection.

3. Play and expressive therapies have a unique kinesthetic quality. Expressive media provide this unique sensory experience, and meet the need that all persons have for kinesthetic experiences. This is a fundamental reality that is an extension of basic attachment needs, which is met through experience and relationship.

4. Play and expressive therapies serve to create a necessary therapeutic distance for clients. Clients in emotional crisis are often unable to express their pain in words, but may find expression through a projective medium. It is simply easier for a traumatized client to "speak" through a puppet, a sandtray therapy miniature, or an art creation than to directly verbalize the pain.

5. This therapeutic distance that expressive therapies provides creates a safe place for abreaction to occur. Children, adolescents, and adults who have experienced turmoil and trauma need a therapeutic setting in which to abreact—a place where repressed issues can emerge and be relived—as well as to experience the negative emotions that are often attached.

6. Play and expressive therapies create a place for individual or group clients to experience control. A primary result of trauma or crisis is a loss of control for those in its midst. The loss of emotional, psychological, and even physiological control is one of the most distressing by-products of crisis and conflict. Clients in turmoil feel the frustration and fear of having lost control. A crucial goal for these clients must be to empower them, following any personal or family trauma that has been disempowering.

7. Play and expressive therapies naturally provide boundaries and limits, which in turn promotes safety for clients. Boundaries and limits define the therapeutic relationship, as well as any other relationship. Sweeney (1997) suggested: "A relationship without boundaries is not a relationship; rather, it is an unstructured attempt at connection that cannot be made because the people have no specific rules for engagement. A world without limits is not a safe world, and children do not grow where they do not feel safe" (p. 103).

8. Play and expressive therapies naturally provide unique settings for the emergence of therapeutic metaphors. It can be argued that the most powerful metaphors in therapy are those that are generated by clients themselves. Expressive therapy creates an ideal setting for this to occur. The toys and expressive media facilitate clients expressing their own therapeutic metaphors.

9. Play and expressive therapies are effective in overcoming client resistance. Children generally do not self-refer, and not all group or individual clients are enthusiastic about entering therapy. Expressive therapies, because of their non-threatening and engaging qualities, can captivate and draw in the involuntary or reticent client.

10. Play and expressive therapies provide a needed and effective communication medium for the client with poor verbal skills. In addition to the developmental importance of providing children with a nonverbal medium of communication, there are clients of all ages who have poor verbal skills, for a variety of reasons.

This includes clients who experience developmental language delays or deficits, those with social or relational difficulties, physiological challenges, etc.

11. Conversely, play and expressive therapies can cut through verbalization that is used as a defense. For the pseudo-mature child or the verbally sophisticated adult, who may use rationalization and/or intellectualization as defenses, expressive therapies can cut through these defenses. This is an important dynamic to be aware of, because an individual or group that presents as verbally well-defended may also include one or more members unable to establish effective communication and relationship.

12. The challenge of transference may be effectively addressed through play and expressive therapies. The presence of an expressive medium creates an alternative object of transference. Regardless of one's theoretical view of transference, however, expressive therapies provide a means for transference issues to be safely addressed as needed. The expressive media can become objects of transference as well as the means by which transference issues are safely addressed.

13. Play and expressive therapies are effective interventions for traumatized clients. There are neurobiological effects of trauma (including prefrontal cortex dysfunction, over-activation of the limbic system, and deactivation of the Broca's area [part of the brain responsible for speech]) that point to the need for nonverbal interventions. The neurobiological inhibitions on cognitive processing and verbalization seem to indicate the benefits of expressive intervention.

14. Lastly, we would argue that deeper intrapsychic and interpersonal issues may be accessed more thoroughly and more rapidly through play and expressive therapies. While access to underlying emotional issues, unconscious conflicts, and interpersonal struggle are challenges for all therapists to address, providing a means for nonverbal expression enables clients a safe means for processing, and often an accelerated one.

Advantages and Rationale for Group Play Therapy

Persons of all ages benefit from the group counseling process. In the same way that talk-based group therapy works with adults, group play therapy works with children, adolescents and adults. One can replace the word *children* in the following quote—from Berg, Landreth, and Fall (2006)—with *adolescents* or *adults*, and it is equally appropriate:

> In group counseling relationships, children experience the therapeutic releasing qualities of discovering that their peers have problems, too, and a diminishing of the barriers of feeling all alone. A feeling of belonging develops, and new interpersonal skills are attempted in a "real life" encounter where children learn more effective ways of relating to people through the process of trial and error. The group then is a microcosm of children's everyday world. In this setting children are afforded the opportunity for immediate reactions from peers as well as the opportunity for vicarious learning. Children also develop a sensitivity to others and receive a tremendous boost to their self-concept through being helpful to

someone else. For abused children who have poor self-concepts and a life history of experiencing failure, discovering they can be helpful to someone else may be the most profound therapeutic quality possible. In the counseling group, children also discover they are worthy of respect and that their worth is not dependent on what they do or what they produce but rather on who they are.

(p. 254)

Clients learn about themselves and others in therapeutic play groups. This is facilitated because the expressive play process promotes communication. Thus, they learn as they observe and listen to the group play therapist and other group members. This is a phenomenological experience, as they perceive the therapist's and other group members' interactions with them. Group members realize that their uniqueness is not just acceptable, it is valued and prized. Egalitarianism and cooperation are promoted and valued in the group play therapy process, and therefore respected. Only when limits need to be set or structured activities are exercised is compliance expected. Creativity and resourcefulness are highly regarded.

Building upon the above rationale for play therapy, there is a specific rationale for employing group play therapy. Sweeney (1997, 2011a) and Sweeney and Homeyer (1999) propose:

1. Groups tend to promote spontaneity in clients of all ages and may, therefore, increase their level of participation in the play or expressive therapy experience. As the therapist attempts to communicate permissiveness, this is further enhanced by the group dynamics, thus freeing clients to risk engagement in various play and relational behaviors.
2. The affective life of group members is dealt with at several levels. First, the intrapsychic issues of individual group members are given opportunity for exploration and expression. Second, both interpersonal and intrapersonal issues are explored—between the therapist and clients, as well as among the clients themselves.
3. Expressive therapy groups provide opportunities for vicarious learning and catharsis. Clients observe the emotional and behavioral expressions of other group members and learn coping behaviors, problem-solving skills, and alternative avenues of self-expression. As clients see other group members engage in activities that they may initially feel cautious or apprehensive about, they gain the courage to explore.
4. Clients experience the opportunity for self-growth and self-exploration in group play therapy. This process is promoted and facilitated by the responses and reactions of group members to a client's emotional and behavioral expression. Clients have the opportunity to reflect and achieve insight to self as they learn to evaluate and reevaluate themselves in light of peer feedback.
5. Play and expressive group therapy provide wonderful and significant opportunities to anchor clients to the world of reality. While most expressions in the play or activity room should be acceptable, limits must be occasionally set and anchors to reality must exist. Limit-setting and reality-testing occur not only between

the therapist and individual group members, but also between group members themselves. The group serves as a tangible microcosm of society; thus, the group play therapy experience is tangibly tied to reality.

6. Since play therapy groups often serve as a microcosm of society, the therapist has the opportunity to gain substantial insight into clients' everyday lives. This "real-life" perspective seen in the microcosm of the playroom can assist with treatment planning and work with family members, teachers, and other significant persons.

7. The group play therapy setting may decrease a client's need or tendency to be repetitious and/or to retreat into fantasy play. While these behaviors may be necessary for some clients in the processing of their issues, the group play therapy setting can bring those clients who are "stuck" in repetition or fantasy into the here and now. This is again accomplished with therapist-initiated interactions and among clients in the group.

8. Clients of all ages have the opportunity to "practice" for everyday life in the group play therapy process. The group provides the opportunity for clients to develop interpersonal skills, master new behaviors, offer and receive assistance, and experiment with alternative expressions of emotions and behavior.

9. The presence of more than one client (or multiple clients) in the play therapy setting may assist in the development of the therapeutic relationship for some clients. As withdrawn or avoidant clients observe the therapist building trust with other clients, they are often drawn in. This helps reduce the anxiety of clients unsure about the play therapy setting and the person of the therapist.

10. Finally, as with therapeutic groups of any kind, group play therapy may provide a more expedient means of intervention in terms of time and expenditure for both clients and family members.

As with most group counseling experiences, the motivation to change is stronger in a group play therapy setting, because the commitment to change is made to more than just a single person. This is part of the experience of commonality, where group members discover not only this motivation, but also the discovery of thoughts and emotions that can be intrapsychically and interpersonally processed. The ability to process through both verbal and nonverbal means is magnified through the expressive and projective nature of the group play therapy experience. We would further contend that these projective and expressive elements further facilitate the crucial sense of belonging that group counseling experiences should inherently foster.

Goals

These rationale point to the goals of group play therapy, because the opportunities for growth and change that are provided for clients in therapeutic play groups are so numerous. Ginott (1961) suggested that group play therapy is based on the assumption that children modify their behavior in exchange for acceptance. We would assert that this applies to adolescents and adults as well. Ginott's premise, combined with the capacity and tendency of clients to seek out and establish relationships, underlies the therapeutic advantage for using group play therapy. Ginott also contended that the primary goal for group play therapy, like all therapy, is enduring personality change (a strengthened ego and enhanced self-image). To this end, he proposes several questions, from which we can summarize the primary therapeutic goals of group play therapy:

1. Does the method facilitate or hinder the establishment of a therapeutic relationship?
2. Does it accelerate or retard evocation of catharsis?
3. Does it aid or obstruct attainment of insight?
4. Does it augment or diminish opportunities for reality testing?
5. Does it open or block channels for sublimation?

(p. 2)

The answers to these questions bring focus to the goals of therapeutic play groups. Group play therapy should facilitate:

1. The establishment of a therapeutic relationship.
2. The expression of emotions.
3. The development of insight.
4. Opportunities for reality testing.
5. Opportunities for expressing feelings and needs in more acceptable ways.

These mirror the goals that Corey (2004) suggests are those shared by members of all group counseling experiences:

- To learn to trust oneself and others
- To increase awareness and self-knowledge; to develop a sense of one's unique identity
- To recognize the commonality of members' needs and problems and to develop a sense of universality
- To increase self-acceptance, self-confidence, self-respect, and to achieve a new view of oneself and others
- To develop concern and compassion for others
- To find alternative ways of dealing with normal developmental issues and resolving certain conflicts
- To increase self-direction, interdependence, and responsibility toward oneself and others
- To become aware of one's choices and to make choices wisely
- To make specific plans for changing certain behaviors and to commit oneself to follow through with these plans
- To learn more effective social skills
- To become more sensitive to the needs and feelings of others
- To learn how to challenge others with care, concern, honesty, and directness
- To clarify one's values and decide whether and how to modify them.

(pp. 5–6)

These should be expected goals in the group play therapy experience, regardless of theoretical orientation and specific group play therapy techniques.

Role of Group Play Therapists

Group play therapists have a crucial role in the functioning and success of the group process. While an "expert," it is generally best to minimize this expert role, and model what is expected and hoped for in the group participants. Clearly stating and then modeling expectations (such as honesty, participation, spontaneity, mutual empathy) will set a tone for the group process. This will, of course, vary according to theoretical perspective and group purpose. Brabender (2002) reminds us: "Beyond the choices that the therapist makes in theoretical frameworks is the person of the therapist, who determines how to interpret his or her role in the group. Group therapists' behavior cannot but be informed by the emotional and cognitive characteristics that they bring to the therapeutic enterprise" (p. 119).

Perhaps most important, however, is the therapist's belief in the process, and communication of this belief to group members. In her chapter on Jungian group play therapy, Bertoia (1999) asserts: "Perhaps the most critical element for success is the therapist—whose belief in the process must be absolute" (p. 102).

The group leader is responsible for identifying and communicating group goals, in a developmentally appropriate manner. The structure, however much structure there is to be, is the responsibility of the group play therapist. This important role does, however, need to be balanced with a forgotten quality for group leaders: patience. Berg et al. (2006) suggest: "Group counseling requires patience and a willingness to allow members to discover for themselves. Patience is indeed a basic prerequisite to the developing of responsibility in a group" (p. 341).

Just as members in a therapeutic play group adapt, as well as collective change in the group community, the role of the leader is adaptive. Group members can and should take on more responsibility, and arguably the group leader should adjust his or her level of control and directiveness. This will depend on the group construction and intent, but as noted earlier, we believe strongly in the group leader being a facilitator. It may be that the group leader's role becomes more of a process monitor. In fact, balancing content and process often becomes the primary role for group leaders as the group moves forward.

This is not to say that as group members take on more responsibility that group leaders abdicate their role of responsibility for the group. Challenging situations often develop in the course of group play therapy, particularly as group members feel a greater sense of safety, and thus express emotion and behavior that may be personally and interpersonally more provocative.

Kottman (2011) discusses the role of the Adlerian play therapist, which applies to both individual and group play therapists. She discusses this in the context of the four stages of Adlerian therapy: (1) the therapist is both partner and encourager; (2) the therapist is an active, relatively directive detective; (3) the therapist is a partner, but also an educator; and (4) the therapist is an active teacher and encourager. These roles accompany many, but not all, approaches to group play therapy.

Also, it is important to note that group play therapy is an *advanced* intervention. It is an intervention that should be practiced by a skilled therapist, with training and supervision in both play therapy and group therapy. Ray (2011) summarizes this important dynamic:

> Group play therapy employs the advanced skills of experienced play therapists. Individual play therapy allows the therapist the freedom to control many variables of the therapeutic process. The therapist sets the environment and makes decisions regarding how to respond to the individual child. Interactions are often predictable because the therapist anticipates how each of his responses will be received by the child. However, the modality of group play therapy requires that the therapist accept the inevitability of human contact over which the therapist has no control. Group play therapy demands not only the expertise of the therapist in play therapy, but also an expertise in facilitation and a secure level of acceptance with the interactions of others. Group play therapy offers a challenging environment for play therapists by requiring a comfort level with positive and negative interactions that take place between children, commitment to the belief that children can be therapeutic agents for each other, and additional skills beyond what is expected of a play therapist in individual therapy. The confidence of a play therapist is sometimes shaken by the mere increase in activity levels that occurs in group therapy when compared to individual play therapy. Play therapists may also have reactions to perceived lack of control, the inability to be therapeutic in response giving, and a reduced feeling of intimacy with clients that was experienced in individual therapy. To overcome these challenges and reactions, a play therapist will need to embrace the value of the group method, recognizing its effectiveness for therapy over individual methods in specific cases.
>
> (pp. 183–184)

Group Play Therapy and Evidence-Based Practice

Chapter 15 will address research in the field of group play therapy. It is important, however, to make a few brief comments here about evidence-based practice (EBP). Our first comment is that it is important to understand the term evidence-based practice, a term that is occasionally misunderstood. In 2006, the APA established a task force on EBP in psychology. This task force (American Psychological Association Presidential Task Force on Evidence-Based Practice, 2006) attempted to establish varying types of clinical research evidence and stated this definition: "Evidence-based practice in psychology is the integration of the best available research with clinical expertise in the context of patient characteristics, culture, and preferences" (p. 273).

We fully support EBP, which is one of the reasons we have included a chapter on research in this book. A challenge exists, however, when EBP is misused or when existing research is not acknowledged as evidence-based. One manner in which EBP is misused is when a study with one population is used to justify using the same intervention with another. For example, if a particular intervention is used with a particular diagnosis with a particular developmental age, it is inappropriate to call the intervention EBP when used with a different diagnosis and/or with a different developmental age. This is not EBP, nor is it *empirically informed*, another term that is occasionally misused.

Also, it needs to be pointed out that an intervention that is not yet researched or has not been researched with a larger population may indeed not qualify as an EBP. However, unproven does not mean ineffective. We make this point not to argue for non-EBP interventions, nor to justify using interventions that are on the fringe of acceptability. We support EBP. There is research on group play therapy. We do have concerns about the misunderstanding of EBP, however.

Group play therapy is an exciting intervention, and needs experienced therapists, as well as further research. Axford and Morpeth (2013) make the point: "It should also be noted that if a suitable program does not exist it is unhelpful to impose one that is unsuitable. Indeed, a central tenet of the evidence-based practice approach is that conclusive evidence of effectiveness may not exist and the choice of intervention might need to be based on the best evidence available, a practitioner's theoretical knowledge or their experience of what works with their population" (p. 274).

Conclusion

Group play therapy is not for the faint of heart. The role requires training, supervised experience, belief in the process, and courage. Group play therapy has been successfully employed with children, adolescents, and adults for some time. While it has been somewhat underutilized, we are excited about the successful blending of play therapy and group process. Clients grow in a setting and process that helps them translate their learning into life outside of the play setting (Sweeney & Homeyer, 1999). Groups serve as a practice field for the outside world, and the expressive and projective nature of group play therapy enables this practice to become real, thus easier to transfer into interpersonal and intrapersonal functioning.

2   Theoretical Approaches to Group Play Therapy

Typically, therapists operate from a theoretical approach to facilitate group play therapy. Operating from a clear theoretical rationale in working with clients provides counselors with "an explanation of how each person was innately endowed and developed throughout one's lifetime so far" (Fall, Holden, & Marquis, 2010, p. 2). In addition, comprehensive theory offers explanation of problems faced by people and a description of dynamics or conditions for change. Providing group play therapy from a specific theoretical approach offers direction for the counselor in treatment planning. By understanding and conceptualizing children in a way that addresses their development, thoughts, feelings, and behavior, a therapist can determine therapeutic goals and most effective practice to reach those goals. Theoretically-driven practice serves as a roadmap for the counselor to operative consistently and effectively.

Play therapy is a modality approached from a range of diverse theoretical orientations. As with most therapeutic modalities, the roots of group play therapy are within the psychoanalytic framework. Child-centered play therapy (CCPT) is recognized as the most popular approach to play therapy in the United States, with cognitive behavioral play therapy (CBPT) and Adlerian play therapy (AdPT) as distant second and third orientations in use by practitioners (Lambert et al., 2005). Gestalt and Jungian play therapy orientations have been addressed extensively in the literature and their use with group play therapy modalities explored. Additionally, literature on Ecosystemic play therapy has addressed the use of group play therapy. The purpose of this chapter is to briefly introduce the basics of each theoretical orientation and its approach to group play therapy. Theories addressed in this chapter include theories in the literature that have explored group play therapy as a direct service to children. Hence, theories or modalities that involve group approaches for parents are not included (i.e., filial play therapy, Theraplay®). For each theory, we will provide a brief synopsis of developmental constructs, therapeutic approach, and considerations for group play therapy. Readers are encouraged to further review these approaches with rigor, noting that a thorough analysis of these approaches is beyond the scope of this book.

Psychoanalytic Play Therapy

The beginnings of play therapy are traced back to Sigmund Freud (1909/1955), who never directly worked with children but described the case of "Little Hans," a child who had developed a phobia, refusing to leave the house due to his fear of being bitten by a horse. S. Freud directed Hans' father to observe and report Hans' play behavior to Freud, who then analyzed the boy through correspondence. Melanie Klein (1975/1932) and Anna Freud (1946) were credited with the expansion of play therapy through their exploration, writings, and presentation on play as a method for psychoanalysis. Psychoanalytic play therapy offered the first organized approach to play therapy, providing a theoretical rationale and description of practice.

Developmental Constructs

S. Freud (1949) introduced the structural model of personality development that consisted of three structures, the id, ego, and superego. The id is the entire personality of the infant and the source of all energy for personality development (Fall et al., 2010). The id, sitting entirely in the unconscious, operates entirely from the pleasure principle by seeking to avoid pain. The id is the home to instinctual drives and operates without rationality. The ego is the structure that develops as a result of the id's interaction with the real world. As the ego develops, it realizes that in order to meet the needs of the id in reality, gratification may be delayed or denied. In the process, the ego helps the development of a personal sense of self for each person. The superego develops as the internal judge of the self, developed from the internalization of ideals from the external world, mainly parents (A. Freud, 1946). Because the superego operates from the place of ideals, it is also considered irrational and often a harsh master of the ego.

Within the structural model, the purpose of a person is to satisfy innate biological needs, the need to fulfill the pleasure principle (Lee, 2009). Needs inspire the development of drives, which are experienced as disturbing tensions that a person seeks to release through imagination or action (Fall et al., 2010). The negotiation of drives in the context of reality, as played out by the id, ego, and superego, is what guides personality development.

Freud was one of the first developmental theorists to offer a model for use by all therapists, but seems especially salient for child therapists. Lee (2009) emphasized that the process of development through the fulfillment of the pleasure principle and negotiation of structures is most clearly seen in early childhood. Freud identified five stages of development: oral, anal, phallic, latent, and genital. The compromise of drives within reality during these stages results in healthy development or maladjustment. In the oral stage, the first stage of infancy, pleasure centers on the mouth and derives from activities involving the mouth, such as sucking, eating, and biting. Unsuccessful attempts at meeting this need may result in dependency or defiant independence (Fall et al., 2010). During the anal stage, which occurs after the first year of life, the focus is on the anus with the chief task being toilet training. When the drive is met through effective attempts to retain and release feces, the child is learning self-control and regulation. In the phallic stage, around three to five years of age, the child becomes focused on genitals leading to the Oedipus complex, resolution of which determines the person's approach to sexuality. From approximate ages of 6 to 11 years, a child enters the latency stage, which is a stage marked by a focus on outside socialization and an absence of a psychosexual emphasis. As puberty emerges, the person enters the genital phase where he or she will remain throughout adulthood. The focus and drive is on sexuality regarding self and other, as well as reproduction. For the child therapist, therapy is typically occurring during one of the early stages of development, hence their importance in psychoanalytic play therapy.

Therapeutic Approach

Lee (2009) eloquently presented the goal of psychoanalytic play therapy: "The ultimate goal of child analysis is to explore, understand, and resolve the etiology of the arrests, fixations, regressions, defensive operations, and so forth, which bind up important sources of psychic energy to aid the resumption of normal development" (p. 43). Psychoanalytic play therapy originated the nondirective approach in child therapy. Extending from the emphasis on free association in psychoanalysis, nondirectivity in play therapy allows the child to choose toys, games, materials, and actions in play, as well as setting the direction and intensity of play (Lee, 2009). Psychoanalytic play therapy highlights the therapeutic value of play itself. Slavson and Schiffer (1975) explained that play can be used as an abreactive ego defense, provides fantasy to cope with limitations of reality, and allows symbolic expression of conflicts.

Klein (1975/1932) recognized the value of play in therapy due to the child's ability to show immediate representations of experiences and fixations through the use of play. Klein believed that play was the child form of free association and interpreted everything done in play as having an underlying symbolic function. She also suggested that children have the insight necessary to recognize the meaning of their behaviors if pointed out by the therapist. A. Freud (1946) differed from Klein in that she did not believe that interpretations of child's play were valuable without the transference relationship necessary for analysis. She proposed that children needed a preparatory period for analysis in which the therapist establishes the transference relationship. The transference relationship is still considered the most effective component of psychoanalytic play therapy. As the therapist offers self as the transitional object, the child will enact the themes and issues with which the child is struggling (Lee, 2009). Level and frequency of interpretation of the transference relationship or the play itself varies among psychoanalytic play therapists. Some feel that interpretation is valuable and can create insight for the child, while others feel that children benefit more from the nondirective play in a safe relationship free from the pressure of what might be confusing interpretations.

Considerations for Group Play Therapy

Literature on psychoanalytic play therapy was the first to address group play therapy and provide a clear structure for its delivery (Ginott, 1961). Slavson and Schiffer (1975) identified elements of group play therapy that make it the preferred modality over individual therapy. These elements included: (1) it enables therapists to treat large numbers of children; (2) through stimulation by others, children perceive, learn, and utilize different methods of play; (3) it makes the young child more conscious of others; (4) children grow in the realization that a child's pleasure-seeking urges must be accommodated to the needs of others; (5) it provides a psychological miniature setting within which reality-testing can take place; and (6) children become consciously aware of similarities with others.

Establishing and maintaining an effective transference relationship between therapist and child is still a primary objective, even in group play therapy. The therapist operates in a nondirective manner, remaining more of an observer than a participant. The role of observer allows the therapist to develop insight into the children and respond with accurate interpretations. However, due to the nature of group dynamics, the therapist will often intervene to respond to children's questions or conflict between children. Therapists may also interact in the children's play if requested, but must still follow the child's lead to remain as nondirective as possible (Slavson & Schiffer, 1975).

Psychoanalytic play therapists recommend as much freedom as possible in group play therapy (Ginott, 1961; Slavson & Schiffer, 1975). Limit-setting is infrequent and only provided when necessary, such as limiting aggressive acts between children. Because of the level of freedom provided in group play therapy, the therapist must remain vigilant and anticipate problematic interactions. Due to the need for free expression, psychoanalytic play therapy allows for a variation of play materials, including materials that are considered nurturing, aggressive, and fantasy.

The focus of group play therapy is always the individual child (Ginott, 1961). Children are free to play independently or with each other. As in individual play therapy, the therapist follows the children as individuals throughout the session. If there are group goals or group rules, they are set by group members, not by the therapist. The mere presence of other children and probable ensuing interaction between children and therapist are considered to be the therapeutic factors of group play therapy.

Child-Centered Play Therapy (CCPT)

CCPT was developed in the 1940s, distinguishing it as one of the longest-standing mental health interventions used today. Based on Rogers' (1951) person-centered theory, Virginia Axline (1947) presented the first structure of CCPT by operationalizing the philosophy of person-centered therapy into a coherent working method for children. Axline referred to this approach as nondirective play therapy, which was later termed child-centered play therapy. In the years since the introduction of CCPT, 62 outcome studies have confirmed its effectiveness, resulting in CCPT being the most researched of all play therapies (Ray, 2011).

Developmental Constructs

In his explanation of person-centered theory, Rogers (1951) introduced 19 propositions to explain personality development and behavior. The 19 propositions provide a framework for human development and explain in great detail how maladjustment in the human condition occurs. These propositions also provide the rationale for CCPT intervention and serve as a guide for play therapists in understanding and facilitating the change process (Ray, 2011). According to Rogers, the human response to experience is organic and holistic, forward moving, and striving for enhancement of the organism (organism is the term used by Rogers to describe the individual person). The essential concept for growth and change is that personality development lies in the phenomenological experience of the organism. In more simplistic terms, specifically regarding children, a child is born into the world viewing interactions in a unique and personal way that is apart from reality or others' perceptions. However, the child will move holistically toward what is most enhancing for the self-organism.

The development of the self is separate from the phenomenological field, but is also highly influenced by it. One eventually comes to evaluate self-worth based upon the perceived expectations and acceptance of others (termed "conditions of worth"). Conditions of worth eventually integrate into the developing self, so that subsequent experiences represent one's internalized representations of how he or she is valued. Thus, a sense of self is established through interactions with significant others and the child's perceptions of those interactions. A child's interactions result in an attitude of self-worth that is influenced by a perceived sense of acceptance by and expectations of others. If a child feels unworthy or unaccepted for certain aspects of self, this sets up barriers for self-acceptance. Behavior is seen as an attempt to maintain the organism and have one's needs met depending upon the perceived expectations of the environment, while the emotion accompanying behavior is seen as dependent on the perceived need for behavior. Hence, a child will behave and emotionally respond in a way that is consistent with the view of self, even if the view of self does not facilitate the optimal growth of the individual. More concretely, if a child feels unaccepting of self or unaccepted by others, feelings and behaviors will be more negative and less self-enhancing.

Therapeutic Approach

There are six postulated conditions that must exist in order for the child-centered therapeutic process to work effectively. All six conditions are based on the primacy of the relationship between therapist and child. They include (1) two persons are in psychological contact; (2) the first person (client) is in a state of incongruence; (3) the second person (therapist) is congruent in the relationship; (4) the therapist experiences unconditional positive regard for client; (5) the therapist experiences an empathic understanding of the client's internal frame of reference and attempts to communicate this experience to the client; and (6) communication to the client of the therapist's empathic understanding and unconditional positive regard is to a minimal degree achieved (Rogers, 1957).

Similar to psychoanalytic play therapy, CCPT is characterized by a nondirective attitude toward play sessions. However, nondirectivity in CCPT is utilized for a different purpose in that it is an attitude that promotes the child's self-sufficiency by not guiding the client's goals or therapeutic content (Ray, 2011). The child leads what is said and done in a play session. Axline (1947) offered guidelines to enact the philosophy of nondirectivity in the context of the CCPT structure. They are referred to as the 8 Basic Principles, which are paraphrased below:

1. The therapist develops a warm, friendly relationship with the child as soon as possible.
2. The therapist accepts the child exactly as is, not wishing the child were different in some way.
3. The therapist establishes a feeling of permissiveness in the relationship so that the child can fully express thoughts and feelings.
4. The therapist is attuned to the child's feelings and reflects those back to the child to help gain insight into behavior.

5. The therapist respects the child's ability to solve problems, leaving the responsibility to make choices to the child.
6. The therapist does not direct the child's behavior or conversation. The therapist follows the child.
7. The therapist does not attempt to rush therapy, recognizing the gradual nature of the therapeutic process.
8. The therapist sets only those limits that anchor the child to reality or make the child aware of responsibilities in the relationship.

(pp. 73–74)

These principles provide the structure for play therapy, encouraging the therapist to accept, trust, and follow the child. Although the therapist seeks to avoid leading the child, CCPT is characterized by a high level of relational interaction between therapist and child in which the therapist provides statements of reflection, encouragement, self-responsibility, and limits when necessary. The therapist also responds to the child's direction by participating in play when requested. CCPT is conducted in a playroom stocked with toys that encourage the expression of all feelings by a child. Materials for the playroom include toys, craft materials, paints, easel, puppet-theater, sand box, and child furniture.

Considerations for Group Play Therapy

Group play therapy presents the individual child with an opportunity to express personal strengths and challenges related to self-regard in the presence of other children who will provide feedback, acceptance, and hopefully, support (Ray, 2011). Through the group process, each child is able to build congruence between self-regard and environment in a microcosm of a typical childhood setting where peers are generally present and interactive. The play therapist provides an environment where group members choose direction for self and group, knowing that such a setting will lead to a release of the self-actualizing tendency. CCPT allows for full movement and decision-making by each member of the group. For each child present, there are verbal and nonverbal play behaviors, relationships with other children, and relationships with the therapist (Ray, 2011). These behaviors and relationships are manifested in innumerable dynamics happening simultaneously in the playroom. Because of the nature of self-directed activity for each child in group and the need for attunement between therapist and children, a CCPT group typically involves 2–3 children as opposed to larger numbers served from other theoretical orientations (Ray, 2011).

In group play therapy, the therapist does not structure for cohesion between group members. The reason for an individual focus within group is that child-centered group play therapy is grounded in person-centered theory. The group leader models facilitative behaviors including giving autonomy to persons in groups, freeing children for full expression of selves, facilitating learning, stimulating independence, accepting the emerging creativity of the child, delegating full responsibility, offering and receiving feedback, encouraging and relying on self-evaluation, and finding reward in the development and achievement of others (Bozarth, 1998). Each individual child has the innate potential for development of the self-actualizing tendency, leading to a productive approach to self and others. Rogers (1970) believed that group process was much more important than the behavior and statements of the therapist, highlighting the need for attitudinal qualities over concrete therapeutic responses. The therapist may interfere with the process of the group when she feels that she must lead or structure the group to some imagined end goal. Children in group have the ability to be therapeutic for each other in a way that is distinct from the therapist's role. Their approach to each other is one of genuineness and naturally felt empathy, especially when children have experienced similar contexts, personality characteristics, or presenting issues (Ray, 2011).

Cognitive-Behavioral Play Therapy (CBPT)

Although identified as the second most-cited play therapy approach among play therapists (Lambert et al., 2005), CBPT is perhaps the least explored in the context of theoretical orientation. The popularity of the approach appears to be born from overwhelming support of cognitive-behavioral therapy (CBT) with adults. There are multiple cognitive-behavioral approaches, hence conceptualization of child clients becomes challenging. The most consistent contributor to the integration of cognitive-behavioral techniques and a play therapy modality is Susan Knell (1993), who conceptualizes children from Aaron Beck's (1976) cognitive therapy framework. Her additions to CBT using puppets, stuffed animals, books, and toys modify the approach to meet the developmental level of young children.

Developmental Constructs

Beck and Weishaar (2008) described personality as shaped by an interaction between innate characteristics and environment, emphasizing the role of information processing in human responses and adaptation. Each person is susceptible to cognitive vulnerabilities that lead to psychological maladjustment. Psychological distress can be caused by any number of innate, biological, developmental, and environmental factors, but cognitive distortions are the most evident features of maladjustment. However, Knell (2009) points out that there is no personality theory underlying cognitive-behavioral play therapy due to a focus on psychopathology.

There are three major premises of cognitive therapy as described by Knell and Dasari (2011): "(1) thoughts influence the individual's emotions and behaviors in response to events, (2) perceptions and interpretations of events are shaped by the individual's beliefs and assumptions, and (3) errors in logic or cognitive distortions are prevalent in individuals who experience psychological difficulties" (p. 239). Hence, maladaptive distortions are the basis of human behavior and thought, particularly influencing development. Although cognitive distortions may be developmentally appropriate for young children, they can also be maladaptive leading to problematic beliefs or behaviors (Knell & Dasari, 2011).

Therapeutic Approach

CBPT is brief, structured, directive, and problem-oriented within the context of a trusting relationship between child and therapist (Knell, 2009). CBPT is considered to be developmentally sensitive due to its use of play materials and activities. Features of cog-nitive-behavioral play therapy include establishment of goals, selection of play activities, education, and use of praise and interpretations (Knell, 2009). An expected outcome of therapy is that children will modify their maladaptive ideas, leading to less psychopa-thology. In addition to the replacement of maladaptive thoughts is the introduction of adaptive, coping statements by the therapist to help the child improve functioning.

Knell (1994) noted six properties related to the efficacy of CBPT: (1) The child is directly involved in therapy through play; (2) The focus is on the child's thoughts, feelings, fantasies, and environment, not one area exclusively; (3) The child is taught new strategies for coping with situations through adaptive thoughts and behaviors; (4) Therapy is structured, directive, and goal-oriented; (5) Therapy incorporates empiri-cally demonstrated techniques when possible; and (6) Treatment utilizes techniques that can be evaluated empirically.

In CBPT, the process includes the child's shift from negative thoughts to either neu-tral or positive thoughts, therapist teaching the child new coping skills and behaviors, and practice of the new behaviors (Knell & Dasari, 2011). Behavioral techniques such as rewards and praise are used to reinforce adaptive behaviors. Through these pro-cesses, psychopathology is thought to decrease. Techniques are varied but are typically targeted as behavioral or cognitive interventions and should be empirically supported. Play is used to deliver cognitive-behavioral techniques in a way that is understandable to the child and to help the child communicate. A variety of toys and materials are used in CBPT, allowing the child or therapist to choose appropriate materials collaboratively or independently.

The structure of CBPT involves introductory/orientation, assessment, middle, and termination stages (Knell, 1994). In the orientation stage, the therapist works with the parents to introduce the child to play therapy through simple explanation. Dur-ing this stage, the therapist will decide the level of involvement needed by parents. In the assessment stage, the therapist gathers information related to the presenting problem, including interviews, observations, and assessment instruments. During this stage, the therapist develops a treatment plan for the child. In the middle stage, the therapist enacts the treatment plan through the use of play, behavioral, and cognitive techniques. Unstructured and structured play may be used during the middle stage (Knell & Dasari, 2011). Therapy moves into the termination stage when therapeutic goals have been accomplished. The therapist helps prepare the child for termination through explanation and multiple sessions to work through the loss of the therapy rela-tionship and therapy itself.

Considerations for Group Play Therapy

Literature on CBPT has not directly addressed group play therapy from a theoretical perspective. Many child interventions based on CBT integrate the use of toys or play materials to deliver curriculum to small and large groups of children. However, they typically do not identify as CBPT interventions. Due to CBPT's incorporation of edu-cation, focus on problem-solving, and use of play only as a means to communicate, it seems plausible that there are innumerable interventions that could identify as CBPT. Fischetti (2010) listed several CBT curriculums that utilize play in group formats to address anger management, while Blundon and Schaefer (2006) presented a social skills play group based on cognitive-behavioral strategies. Reddy (2012) provided social skills sequences and interventions designed to teach pro-social skills through group play.

Among the multiple references to CBT, child play therapy and group play therapy, there seem to be some common factors. Each of the interventions that incorporate aspects of CBT and group play therapy emphasizes the educational components of the intervention. In the CBPT approach to groups, a structured educational curriculum seems common. Additionally, the interventions incorporate traditional behavioral techniques such as positive reinforcement and modeling to support what is being taught in the curriculum. Although in individual CBPT, Knell presented the need for a variety of toys and materials, group approaches to CBPT appear to limit materials to those necessary for the structured activities, eliminating the requirement of a traditional playroom. Yet, individual and group approaches to CBPT both continue to focus on the assimilation of adaptive thoughts in place of maladaptive distortions and negative behaviors.

Adlerian Play Therapy (AdPT)

When play therapists were surveyed, participants noted Adlerian play therapy as the third most identified theory in use (Lambert et al., 2005). Terry Kottman is noted as the founder of AdPT. Although the Adlerian theoretical approach of Individual Psychology was widely known and Adlerian philosophy had influenced child guidance centers and theories of child development for almost a century (Mosak & Maniacci, 2008), Kottman (2003) was the first to formalize Adlerian principles into a comprehensive methodology for play therapy. Additionally, she has written extensively on adapting AdPT to the group modality.

Developmental Constructs

Adlerian theory proposes that people are born with an innate capacity to connect with others (Kottman, 2010). This concept of social interest was defined by Fall et al. (2010) as "the motivation to strive for superiority in a way that contributes constructively to others and to society" (p. 106). The development of social interest serves as a marker of mental health. Two further concepts from Individual Psychology serve as the basis to understanding human development. Adler believed in the concepts of phenomenology, an individual's perception of experience was reality for that person, and holism, the view that mind and body work together for a unified personality (Fall et al., 2010).

The central motivation for development in each person is to move from a natural state of inferiority to superiority, causing an individual to develop a lifestyle that organizes experiences. Each person's unique lifestyle is based on interaction with others, perception of experiences, and observation (Kottman, 2010). As children interact with the environment, they creatively develop strategies to find a sense of significance (Fall et al., 2010). Behavior is a manifestation of this lifestyle and response to immediate environmental demands (Mosak & Maniacci, 2008). Hence, all behavior is purposeful, serving the individual lifestyle of the person and the life goals related to that lifestyle.

The lifestyle, complete with life goals, personal private logic, and purposeful behavior, is developed by the age of five or six years.

Kottman (2009) summarized four factors related to personality development according to Adlerian theory. People have an innate need to belong and gain significance, emphasizing the social embeddedness of each person. People move toward goals. In order to understand the person, one must understand the goal of the person's behavior. People are creative and can use their creativity to move toward goal attainment. And finally, people experience life from a subjective perspective, interpreting experiences in a unique way as they go through life.

Therapeutic Approach

Kottman (2009) offered seven goals of Adlerian play therapy, helping the client (a) gain an awareness of and insight into lifestyle; (b) alter faulty self-defeating apperceptions and move from private logic to common sense; (c) move toward positive goals of behavior; (d) replace negative strategies for belonging and gaining significance with positive strategies; (e) increase his or her social interest; (f) learn new ways of coping with feelings of inferiority; and (g) optimize creativity and begin to use his or her assets to develop self-enhancing decisions about attitudes, feelings, and behaviors (p. 244).

Adlerian play therapists attempt to meet therapeutic goals through several structures, including the four phases of therapy (Kottman, 2010). In the first phase of therapy, the therapist seeks to build an egalitarian relationship with the child through verbal actions such as reflecting, encouraging, and questioning. The therapeutic relationship is the foundation of effective therapy. In the second phase, the therapist explores the child's lifestyle through observation of the child's behavior in the playroom, structured play activities, or questioning. During the third phase, the therapist helps the child gain insight into individual lifestyle by using techniques such as metacommunication, metaphors, storytelling, and structured activities. In the final stage of reorientation and reeducation, the therapist teaches the child new skills and attitudes, as well provides practice opportunities for the child to transfer the skills outside of the playroom.

The Adlerian approach to therapy also addresses helping children work toward positive goals, labeled the Crucial Cs (Kottman, 2010). The therapist helps the child move to feeling connected with others, feeling capable, feeling that they count, and developing courage. As therapy progresses, the therapist notes if the child is struggling in any of these areas and encourages enhancement of these feelings. Encouragement is another key characteristic of the therapist's approach with the child. Adlerian play therapists search for opportunities to encourage children through understanding the lifestyle of each child, connecting with each child, reflecting their care for each child, and providing positive support.

Considerations for Group Play Therapy

Because of emphasis by Adlerian theory on social embeddedness of the person, this particular theory lends itself well to the group play modality. The need to belong as the main goal of the lifestyle indicates that children are likely to respond effectively to group therapy. In group play therapy, Adlerian play therapists are provided with the opportunity to observe children's goals in their interaction with others (Kottman, 1999). Therapists will use problem-solving, facilitating awareness of positive behaviors, and facilitation of feedback from group members to help children improve functioning.

As in individual AdPT, the therapist works to develop a conceptual understanding of each child's lifestyle. Conceptualization is essential to the progression of therapy. Kottman (1999) noted the parallel structure of AdPT to stages of group therapy. In the initial phase, the therapist builds a relationship with each child and facilitates the relationship between children. As the group moves into the transitional stage of group, Adlerian play therapists will use this time to explore the lifestyle of each group member. The third phase of AdPT, facilitating insight into lifestyle, occurs as the group moves into the working stage of group dynamics. In this phase, group members are also gaining insight into each other's lifestyles. During the termination stage of group, AdPT addresses reeducation through providing opportunities for group members to practice skills with each other.

Group play therapy is enhanced by the mix of children who are experiencing different level of difficulties, as well as different abilities. The mix of children helps progression of therapy by utilizing the Adlerian concepts of encouragement and modeling for each other (Kottman, 1999). AdPT for groups may use structured or unstructured approaches, depending on the needs of the group and external pressures such as time limitations. In regard to limit-setting, AdPT utilizes group members to create alternatives and consequences to problems in the playroom. This approach to limit-setting is consistent with the AdPT emphasis by supporting three of the Crucial Cs: helping children feel connected, capable, and significant (count).

Gestalt Play Therapy

Gestalt therapy was founded by Fritz Perls (although he objected to being solely identified as its founder) and is based on philosophical concepts of holism and field theory (Yontef & Jacobs, 2005). Gestalt therapy is a process-oriented therapy concerned with healthy functioning of the whole person including senses, body, emotions, and intellect (Oaklander, 1999). Violet Oaklander (1988) is noted as the founder of Gestalt play therapy and the most prolific author on its use. Gestalt play therapy has influenced the interventions used in many other schools of play therapy due to the experiential nature of its techniques.

Developmental Constructs

The Gestalt understanding of holism asserts that a human is born as a unified whole with interaction between feelings, thoughts, and actions; parts that cannot be separated from one another (Fall et al., 2010). The field theory underpinning Gestalt theory holds that humans can only be understood within the context of which they live. Through the inherent organic process of self-regulation, the person strives to maintain balance between needs and the satisfaction of those needs. All behavior is regulated by the process of organismic self-regulation in which the child experiences needs, causing discomfort, leading the child to take action to satisfy this need by interacting with the environment (Blom, 2006). The satisfaction of the need leads to a state of homeostasis. The continual emergence of needs and success in need fulfillment results in the forward movement toward growth.

Interaction of the child with the environment is called contact and is the core of experience that develops the self, a key concept in Gestalt theory (Carroll, 2009). "Contact is the process of being aware of a need and engaging with the environment in order to fulfill that need, and assimilating the experience for emotional, psychological, or physical growth" (Carroll, 2009, p. 285). It is through this contact that a self emerges that differentiates between me and not-me. Throughout development, the child becomes more active in choosing what is needed or wanted from the environment for healthy functioning. If contact by a child is received as unsupportive or negative to functioning, the child's capacity to self-regulate and engage with the environment becomes constricted. Healthy functioning of a child involves full integration of all aspects of self, with well-being of the child supported externally and internally (Carroll, 2009).

Therapeutic Approach

In Gestalt play therapy, the child needs help to restore healthy self-regulation, become aware of internal and external experiences, and be able to use the environment to get needs met (Carroll, 2009). Blom (2006) clearly stated: "The aim of gestalt play therapy with children is to make them aware of their own process" (p. 51). With awareness, the child perceives a diversity of choices to enable behavioral change for need satisfaction. However, the child needs help to restore healthy self-regulation, develop awareness of internal and external experiences, and be able to use resources in the environment to meet holistic needs (Carroll, 2009).

From the Gestalt perspective, it is the therapist's duty to use multiple methods to "bring out" awareness in a child. Regarding her work with children, Oaklander (1988) wrote: "So it is up to me to provide the means by which we will open doors and windows to their inner worlds. I need to provide methods for children to express their feelings, to get what they are keeping guarded inside out into the open, so that together we can deal with this material" (pp. 192–193). The Gestalt approach emphasizes the need for the child's expression of awareness, often verbally, of the child's world. In addition, the child needs support in experiencing acceptance of parts of self that have been unacceptable (Carroll, 2009). The therapist provides a safe relationship and new experiences that allow the child to experience herself in a new way for the purposes of integration of parts that have previously been denied acceptance.

Oaklander (1988) asserted that most of her techniques used in Gestalt play therapy encouraged projection. Projections facilitate the external expression of the internal self that is rarely displayed. Oaklander recognized that projections may be the only way that some children are willing to disclose their inner thoughts, feelings, and experiences. Interpretations are rarely used in Gestalt play therapy due to their base in the therapist's experience, not the child's. The role of the therapist is to facilitate self-awareness and ownership by the child. The therapist focuses on the process happening with the child and selects techniques accordingly, based on the child and the therapeutic relationship. Gestalt play therapy recognizes the therapist–child relationship as therapeutic in and of itself, and strives to facilitate a relationship of equality and genuineness (Oaklander, 1999).

Considerations for Group Play Therapy

As with most approaches to group play therapy, Gestalt play therapy utilizes the group modality to allow children to operate from present behaviors and try out new behaviors. Oaklander (1999) addressed the process of group from a Gestalt perspective. In the initial phases of group play therapy, the therapist establishes safe and respectful relationships, as well as initiates nonthreatening activities to help group members get to know one another. After 4–6 weeks of group sessions, children start to feel more comfortable through the establishment of support for one another. As children establish individual identities and roles, the therapist will use techniques to bring these roles into awareness. Oaklander recommended that group size consist of 3–6 children for children less than 8 years old and 6–8 children for those who are over 8 years old. The presence of a co-therapist is helpful in addressing the individual needs of some children.

Oaklander further proposed a specific group structure involving an initial round of children reporting what occurred during their week, a structured activity led by the therapist, and then a closing time to allow children to express their thoughts or feelings during the session. The structured activities are usually projective and should facilitate expression of feelings, strengthening of self, and provide an experience to bring out healthier aspects of self. Enjoyment is a key component to Gestalt group play therapy that allows children to move to painful places and subjects while feeling safe and supported.

Jungian Play Therapy

Play therapy, as all modern therapy, began as a psychoanalytic technique, but psychoanalytic play therapy has not retained its popularity among the modality. Interestingly, the Jungian analytical framework emerged as a leading approach to play therapy. Jungian play therapy is the foremost current approach focused on the unconscious processes that occur within the child during the therapeutic process. John Allan (1988) is perhaps the most credited figure in the presentation and organization of Jungian play therapy. His seminal work on play therapy, *Inscapes of the Child's World: Jungian Counseling in Schools and Clinics*, laid the framework for conducting Jungian play therapy, demonstrating its effectiveness in both school and private settings.

Developmental Constructs

From a Jungian perspective, Douglas (2008) explained the personality rests upon the psyche, which is made up of conscious and unconscious components that are tied to the collective unconscious, "underlying patterns of images, thoughts, behaviors, and experiences" (pp. 103–104). Within the collective unconscious lie the archetypes, innate mechanisms of receiving and responding (Allan & Bertoia, 2003). The self is an archetype that strives to grow and make meaning out of existence, yet exists in the unconscious. The ego is a structure inherent at birth as a weak, undifferentiated form but the center of consciousness. As the child grows, the ego mediates between inner drives and external reality (Allan & Bertoia, 2003). Healthy development relies on a good relationship between the self and the ego, the unconscious and the conscious. In healthy people, Allan (1988) clarified that there is a fluid yet regulated connection between the conscious and unconscious. If an infant's needs are not met, there will be breaks in the relationship between self and ego, leading to rigid defenses to protect the fragile ego (Green, 2009).

The central drive in Jungian theory is to establish a separate identity through the individuation process. The constant struggle of opposites that takes place within the person drives the individuation process (Allan & Bertoia, 2003). The language of symbols, including archetypes, dreams, and images, is used to understand the unconscious. The unconscious is a purposeful structure that will move to growth and healing if allowed to be expressed in symbolic form.

Therapeutic Approach

Allan (1997) pointed out that the goal of Jungian play therapy is the activation of the individuation process, which he defined as "helping the child to develop his or her unique identity, to overcome or come to terms with his or her losses or traumas while accepting and adapting to the healthy demands of family, school, and society at large" (p. 105). Green (2009) described the therapist role as an analytic one in which he utilizes directive techniques such as drawings, drama, or sandplay to benefit the exploration of symbols in art interpretation and analysis of transference. These processes allow children to acknowledge unconscious components, integrate into conscious components, and activate the self-healing mechanism available to them. The belief in the role of the child's unconscious processes encourages the Jungian play therapist to directly act upon the child by presenting activities, questioning, and interpreting the child's symbols.

Permissiveness of the therapist toward the child is an essential component of Jungian play therapy. When the child is allowed to express rage or strong conflictual emotions, they can work through these aspects of self to integrate the darker, previously unacknowledged states of being (Green, 2009). Additionally, Jungian play therapy involves the use of symbols through the encouragement of creativity. The use of symbol language activates the child's self-healing archetype and gives expression to the unconscious. Jungian play therapist's work with symbolic expression by asking the child for the meaning of the symbol and asking the child to externalize inner dialogue associated with the symbol (Green, 2009).

Green (2009) summarized that Jungian play therapists "(1) make sense of symbols through an extensive process of personal analysis with a Jungian analyst; (2) conceptualize rage … and help children symbolize it; (3) maintain an analytical attitude that is both involved and detached; (4) possess the ability to direct children's raw material by carrying some of their psychological poison; and (5) use sandplay, artwork, and dream analysis to amplify symbols and follow the child's Self wherever it leads" (p. 91).

Considerations for Group Play Therapy

Both Allan (1988) and Bertoia (1999) presented examples of how Jungian play therapy is applied to small and large groups of children. Allan (1988) described one Jungian group approach in which the counselor opens the group by asking questions about a feeling to stimulate thoughts and feelings, then asking the children to paint, draw, or write a story about that feeling, and closing with children sharing their work with one another. Through this group experience, the children become more aware of their feelings, develop understanding on how to handle their feelings, share feelings with others, communicate their feelings to the counselor, and express their feelings symbolically. Allan believed that the symbolic expression reduced tension and the need for children to act out feelings destructively.

Bertoia (1999) indicated that Jung was not an advocate of groups, seeing them as oppositional to the process of individuation and potentially destructive. However, Bertoia advocated for group play therapy because of the opportunity for interaction of interpersonal relationships with intrapsychic processes that promotes healing. In Jungian play therapy, the therapist begins the process appealing to the conscious level by using clear, rational language and staying in the here and now. The session deepens as the therapist introduces symbolic expression through activity. The therapist closes the session by returning to reality and anchoring the child to the present. In group play therapy, the Jungian therapist attends to the unconscious and the conscious, as well as the personal and collective. By translating the personal and collective images, the therapist helps the group become more aware and move toward healing. Bertoia (1999) believed "it is the therapist's ability for intrapsychic and interpersonal relationship to the personal and collective that determines the outcome" of Jungian group play therapy (p. 102).

Ecosystemic Play Therapy

Ecosystemic play therapy is the approach developed by Kevin O'Connor (1994), which he has continued to refine over the last two decades. Based on systems theory, Ecosystemic theory integrates intrapsychic, interaction, developmental, and historical processes (O'Connor & Ammen, 1997). Ecosystemic play therapy focuses the assessment of and intervention for layers of systems in which the child operates, including family, school, interpersonal relations, culture, intrapsychic understanding, and others. Such a broad perspective toward treatment of children differentiates Ecosystemic play therapy from other approaches. Another unique characteristic of Ecosystemic play therapy is its use as a model that can incorporate many other theoretical orientations but requires the therapist to operate from a consistent personal theory (Kottman, 2010).

Developmental Constructs

Personality development in Ecosystemic play therapy is predicated on the central role of cognitive development and functioning (O'Connor, 2009). Social, moral, and personality development can be limited if cognitive development is limited. Assessment of a child's developmental functioning is essential to case conceptualization and treatment planning. Development beyond biological restraints occurs through the interaction of the child's biological and intrapsychic states and the environment (O'Connor & Ammen, 1997).

From an Ecosystemic perspective, there are three essential elements to personality: "first, that the basic drive motivating human behavior is a derivative of the biologically based survival instinct; second, that the structure and function of personality is inextricably linked to the process of development; and last, that personality derives from the accretion of the residual of one's interactions with the many systems in which one is embedded, that is, one's ecosystem" (O'Connor & Ammen, 1997, p. 9). Due to survival instinct, people are motivated to get their needs met and do so in a variety of ways. Psychopathology occurs when a person cannot get needs met or the attempt to get needs met interferes with the ability of others to get their needs met (O'Connor, 2009). Pathology can occur within the individual due to biological or genetic reasons, through interaction with others when an attempt to get needs met in the context of others is unsuccessful, and/or within a system in which a child is unable to get needs met due to the nature of the system. Repeated engagement in behavior that fails to get the child's needs met and the inability to engage in new ways to get needs met results in need for intervention (O'Connor, 2009).

Therapeutic Approach

O'Connor and Ammen (1997) stated that the primary goal of Ecosystemic play therapy is to help children "get their needs met consistently and in ways that do not interfere with the ability of others to get their needs met" (p. 11). A secondary aim is to facilitate a return to optimal developmental functioning. Ecosystemic play therapy focuses on the individual child, who is seen as operating in three domains: as a physical body; as a child engaging in behavior with the world; and as a child engaging representationally through an internal working model of the world (O'Connor & Ammen, 1997).

The Ecosystemic play therapist engages in two specific strategies: providing the child with corrective experiences and using verbal interventions (O'Connor, 1994). Corrective experiences are provided through symbolic means as the therapist selects materials designed to encourage children to act out options regarding their environment or struggles. Corrective experiences are also initiated through the therapist–child relationship, in which the therapist is in control and uses the control to meet the child's needs. O'Connor (1994) supported the Theraplay® approach that identifies four types of behavior used by the therapist to regulate the child's arousal in session. The first type of behavior is structuring, in which the therapist limits stimulation through behaviors such as preselecting materials or limit-setting. The second behavior is challenging, in which the therapist attempts to increase the arousal level of the child through encouraging a child to do more or go further. The third behavior is intruding, which is also designed to increase arousal. Intruding behaviors prevent the child from withdrawing, and encourage interaction with therapist. The fourth behavior is nurturing and is used to reduce the child's over-arousal and maintain an ideal level of arousal. Nurturing may include physical soothing or verbal reinforcement (O'Connor, 1994).

Verbal interactions are used by the therapist to help the child develop insight into his or her experience. In Ecosystemic play therapy, interpretations are used as the primary tool to facilitate movement towards therapeutic goals. They are effective when they are introduced systematically to the child and in a language that the child understands (O'Connor, 1994). Interpretations range from simple reflective statements to generalizable statements that help a child connect experiences inside session to experiences outside session. Verbal interaction must be balanced with corrective experiences for the most effective outcome to play therapy.

Ecosystemic play therapy holds that play promotes healthy development in children. In therapy, play helps a child to be motivated and engaged, develops a positive relationship between therapist and child, and provides a symbolic tool to link corrective experience, interpretation, and cognitive understanding (O'Connor, 1994). A small number of play materials are carefully selected by the therapist to help provide corrective experiences for the child.

Considerations for Group Play Therapy

Although Ecosystemic play therapy starts with the child's individual functioning, attention is given to systems in which the child operates such as peer and other social groups (O'Connor & Ammen, 1997). Group play therapy offers the opportunity for children to develop strategies to get needs met effectively, a goal of Ecosystemic play therapy (O'Connor, 2009). There is no one Ecosystemic approach to group play therapy. However, O'Connor presented structured group play therapy with the primary purpose of improving the child's interpersonal interactions as one group intervention that fits with the Ecosystemic model (O'Connor, 1999). The group itself provides a corrective experience for the child that is highlighted as a feature of individual treatment.

For structured group play therapy, O'Connor (1999) recommended that children be over the age of five and at similar developmental levels and not experiencing severe psychopathology. Similar to the therapist role in Ecosystemic individual play therapy, the therapist creates and maintains the structure of the group including selecting members, length and duration of treatment, materials, activities, group goals, treatment plan across sessions, as well as maintaining the set structure and ensuring compliance of members. The therapist will also use interpretation to facilitate group members' understanding of the process, which will likely result in member change and generalization of change. In accord with Ecosystemic focus, the therapist provides a group experience that addresses cognitive (problem-solving and interpretation), physical (relaxation training), behavioral (behavior modification system), emotional (guided discussion and interpretation), and social (structured activities) components.

Summary

Each of the theories presented in this chapter represent theoretical approaches that value group play therapy as a viable and necessary intervention. There is consensus among theories that the group modality offers therapists the opportunity to observe and intervene with interpersonal concerns and offers the child the opportunity to practice new ways of being, as well gain relational support. Each theory seeks to facilitate an experience for the child that will encourage the child to develop attitudes and skills that result in interpersonal effectiveness. Additionally, there is agreement that play is the most developmentally appropriate language for the facilitation of therapy. Due to diverse philosophical underpinnings, approaches to group play therapy differ in delivery and style, along with structure and content.

3 Multicultural Issues

Multicultural issues in group play therapy require attention for four reasons. First, the population of U.S. children has changed dramatically in the last decade. The number of children aged 9 years and younger who are other than non-Hispanic White increased by 3,573,000 from the year 2000 to 2009 (U.S. Census Bureau, 2012). Census data show that of the 41,910,000 children aged 9 years and younger in the U.S.A., only 51.4% are non-Hispanic White, 23.8% are Hispanic White, 14.8% are Black, 1.3% are American Indian, 4.7% are Asian, .2% are Hawaiian, and 3.7% are Bi-racial (U.S. Census Bureau, 2012). Since almost half of U.S. children are other than non-Hispanic White, play therapists will likely serve a variety of diverse children in their group play therapy sessions. Play therapists must be just as prepared to serve a group of three White children as a group of one Hispanic, one Black, and one Bi-racial child.

Second, real and perceived differences may exist between children and play therapists. Despite the racial and ethnic diversity of the general population, the diversity of play therapists remains disproportionately low. Approximately 90% of the Association for Play Therapy membership is non-Hispanic White (Bill Burns, personal communication). Economic differences between children and play therapists may also exist. The National Center for Children in Poverty estimates that nearly 44% of American children live in poverty. The percentage of play therapists living in poverty is likely to be far less. These racial, ethnic, and economic differences between children and play therapists require play therapists to be diligent in understanding differing world views, family values, play behavior, experiences of discrimination, parenting practices, etc. For example, a White play therapist gaining the trust of a Black parent may take considerably more time than if the parent was White.

Third, play therapists have an ethical obligation to develop cultural competence and respect individual differences. The codes of ethics that address multicultural issues include the American Counseling Association (A.2.c Developmental and Cultural Sensitivity, A.4.b Personal Values, C.5 Nondiscrimination), the National Association of Social Workers (1.05 Cultural Competence and Social Diversity; 4.02 Discrimination), and the American Psychological Association (2.01 b Boundaries of Competence, 3.01 Unfair Discrimination). Based on these codes of ethics, multicultural issues include race, ethnicity, national origin, color, sex, sexual orientation, gender identity or expression, age, marital status/partnership, political belief, religion, language preference, immigration status, socioeconomic status, or mental or physical disability. The

Association for Play Therapy (APT) Best Practices also states that play therapists do not discriminate on the aforementioned characteristics. Furthermore, APT (2009) Best Practices state:

> Play therapists will actively participate in the provision of interventions that show understanding of the diverse cultural backgrounds of their clients, being cognizant of how their own cultural/ethnic/racial identity may influence interventions and therapeutic philosophy. The play therapist should make every effort to support and maintain the culture and cultural identity of clients.
>
> (p. 3)

Therefore, play therapists must maintain adherence to ethical code and integrity of the play therapy profession by attending to multicultural issues. In fact, play therapists are obligated to confront and educate play therapists who treat children with a color-blind approach (i.e., not honoring and adapting to cultural differences).

Fourth, group dynamics will be impacted by cultural differences, particularly in the perception of power, boundaries, roles, norms, sense of belonging, linking, responding to prejudice, etc. (McRae & Short, 2010). Groups reflect the dynamics of a larger social, cultural, and racial context in which they are imbedded. Many of these racial-cultural group dynamics are unconscious, even to the play therapist. Thus, to respond effectively, play therapists must not only be aware of how these dynamics impact children but also develop multiculturally competent skills.

Multicultural Competence

Multicultural competence for mental health professionals was framed by D. W. Sue et al. (1982) as having the following three components: (a) attitudes and beliefs—awareness of one's own assumptions, values, and biases; (b) knowledge—understanding the worldview of culturally diverse clients; and (c) skills—developing appropriate intervention strategies and techniques. Multicultural awareness, knowledge, and skills are not a onetime acquisition but rather require ongoing study and dedication. Hence, play therapists need to revisit these three components for each and every new child in the playroom.

Awareness

Awareness of one's own culture including world view, meanings, values, rituals, and daily behavior is the beginning of multicultural competence (Sue et al., 1982). Recognizing how one's own cultural aspects differ for diverse populations will decrease unconscious impositions of values and beliefs onto clients and increase empathy and the therapeutic relationship (Gil & Drewes, 2005). Some expression of cultural values and beliefs are inadvertently offensive to differing populations. A well-intended question "what did you get for Christmas?" may be offensive to children who are Muslim, while a question "where does your dad work?" may be offensive to children of lesbians.

Self-awareness. Play therapists can facilitate awareness of their own cultural identity through expressive art projects such as drawing a family crest with symbols of cultural identity or playing a game of cultural card sorting. Exposure to different cultures, whether through travel or reading, can also reveal dearly held values and beliefs while increasing appreciation for others' culture. For example, while visiting a small village in Tanzania, I (Baggerly) noticed a 3-year-old boy following me during a 10-minute walk. When I expressed concern that he was not with his parents, my travel guide smiled and said "Everyone in the village knows him and takes care of him wherever he is." I realized the people in the Tanzanian village had a collectivist view of childcare, while I had an individualist view of childcare. This realization prevented me from judging the child as misbehaving and the family as being neglectful. Rather, I had a new appreciation for the social wealth of this child and family, despite the fact that they lived in economic poverty.

Awareness of cultural issues. In group play therapy, awareness of how racially or ethnically diverse children experience the play therapy process should also be examined. Play therapists may assume the play therapy room is safe for all children. Yet, some children may judge others by the color of their skin rather than the content of their character. One child within the group may be subtly left out by others of a different race. Dynamics of racism, sexism, heterosexism, classism, nationalism, religious prejudice, etc. could be subtly played out without recognition. Consider this interaction between Aaron, a 6-year-old non-Hispanic White from an affluent family and Jose, a 5-year-old recent Mexican immigrant whose family is undocumented.

AARON: Let's play cops and robbers. I'm the cop, you're the robber, and I chase you.

JOSE: No, I don't like that game. (Has a hesitant look on his face and turns toward the sand box).

AARON: If you don't play with me then I'm going to tell on you! Now, turn around, you're under arrest. (Sticks a toy gun in his back and grabs his hands to handcuff).

Clearly, Jose would not view this playroom as a safe environment. The play therapist must intervene to promote a sense of safety immediately after Juan's initial decline. The play therapist could reflect feelings and returning responsibility as follows.

PLAY THERAPIST: Jose, you are uncomfortable with that particular game. Sometimes that game can be scary for some kids. Aaron, you can choose another game to play with Jose or play with him in the sand box.

This type of response that addresses both boys would likely redirect them into a different activity. However, if Aaron continued with the next comment, the play therapist would need to protect Jose with therapeutic limit-setting, such as:

PLAY THERAPIST: Aaron, I know you really want to play cops and robbers, but Jose said he did not want to play that. You can choose to see if he wants to play another game or you can play with something else. Jose, you can choose to tell him what you would like to do.

This response communicates a social boundary that forcing someone is not acceptable. It also communicates that each child has his own voice and each voice is honored.

Awareness of Group Process.   Each play therapist must increase personal awareness of how his or her personal experiences with diverse people may influence the group play therapy process (Gil & Drewes, 2005). This begins with a thorough reflection of one's first exposure to people of a different race, economic level, religion, ability level, etc. Remembering one's own emotions, thoughts, and conclusions helps prevent counter-transference onto children in the playroom. For example, I (Baggerly) have an uncle who is blind. My childhood memories of Uncle Tom were playing with him in the swimming pool, listening to him play the guitar, and hearing him give detailed facts during a tour of Washington, D.C. I feel fondness toward him, believe he is smart, and concluded that people who are blind can do many exciting things. When asked if a child who is blind can be in group play therapy with a child who is sighted, I respond "of course!" In contrast, if another play therapist's early memory was going to a nursing home to visit an elderly relative who was blind, then her emotions may have been uneasiness and she may have concluded people who are blind are incapable. As a result, she may not include a child who is blind in group play therapy or may be overprotective in her therapeutic responses.

Mitigating biases.   When biases or uneasiness is identified, play therapists can seek new information, experiences, or relationships to reformat these limiting schemas. Attending community events, meeting diverse people, and listening to others' stories may help play therapists integrate new perceptions into their schema. Continuing with the example, a play therapist could contact the Lighthouse for the Blind to find a local community event where he could interact with families who have children who are blind. Asking parents to describe how their children play with other children may bring new insight that will lead to more therapeutic responses in group play therapy such as returning responsibility.

Play therapy supervision is essential to increase awareness of cultural biases that play therapists may not recognize. Since supervisees cannot report biases of which they are unaware, supervisors need to view video tapes of group play therapy sessions. For example, while supervising one of my students' group play therapy sessions at the homeless shelter, I noticed she had an unusual response to two children named Tasha and Cathy.

Tasha: Here Cathy, put the food on the table so we can eat dinner.

Cathy: Oh there doesn't look like there is enough food for all of us!

Tasha: You know there never is! Now give her [pointing to the play therapist] some food. I just won't eat.

Play therapist: Tasha, you want me to eat but you can have my food. I don't need that much.

During supervision, I replayed the segment of video twice and asked the play therapist what she noticed about her voice tone and response. She admitted that it was rapid and higher pitched than usual and that her response did not allow the child to lead the play. I asked her to identify her feelings, thoughts, and motivations during the play session. While reflecting on her feelings, the play therapist realized her anxiety was rooted in her own childhood experiences of poverty and having to share food with relatives who did not have enough. When asked how this may have impacted the group dynamics, the play therapist realized the children may have sensed her anxiety and altered their play reenactment, as well as potential resolution, due to their embarrassment or need to protect her. To the play therapist's credit, she spent time journaling and speaking with relatives about their experience to mitigate the intensity of her experience with poverty.

Knowledge

In addition to increasing awareness, group play therapy effectiveness is enhanced by building knowledge about diversity. Group play therapists need to know how to obtain cultural knowledge without stereotyping. One helpful acronym that prevents stereotyping and shows the complexity of all people is RESPECTFUL (Ivey, D'Andrea, Ivey, & Simek-Morgan, 2006). These letters represent:

Religion/Spirituality
Economic Class
Sexual Orientation
Psychological Maturity
Ethnic/Racial Identity
Chronological Challenges/Age
Trauma
Family History
Unique Physical Characteristics
Language and Location of Residency.

These ten varying characteristics accentuate the uniqueness of each child in a group, even if they are the same race. For example, two Black boys may be in a group. One boy may be a Black Cuban immigrant from a lower socioeconomic Miami neighborhood who speaks Spanish and is Catholic. The other boy may be a Black African American from an upper middle class New York City neighborhood whose parents converted to Islam. Kotchick and Forehand (2002) also emphasize that children's and parents' cultural characteristics are mitigated within group contextual factors such as individual temperament and family financial standing. For example, they report urban African American parents with a low income tend to be more controlling and less affectionate than African American parents with a higher income. Kotchick and Forehand postulate this parenting practice of the former is an adaptive response of teaching children how to be independent in a dangerous situation.

Cultural norms. Since each child has unique characteristics as reflected in the RESPECTFUL acronym, it is unwise to automatically apply a list of cultural characteristics to a child. However, knowing some cultural norms of various groups will provide a context in which to begin to understand within-group differences a particular child may experience. For example, as a whole, Asian students tend to do better academically than non-Asian students. In 2009, 48% of Asian fourth grade students in Texas scored proficient or higher in reading compared with only 16% of African Americans, 20% of Latinos, and 44% of Whites (Education Trust, 2009). This fact that Asians as a whole are "smart" in school provides a context in which to understand Yu-fen, a Taiwanese American fourth grade girl who has a reading disability. She suffers from low self-esteem, partly due to other children in group play therapy who perpetuate the stereotype that "Asians are supposed to be smart."

Yu-fen: I can't read this book.

Eric: All Asians are supposed to be smart, why aren't you?

Play Therapist: Eric, you are surprised but not all people of one ethnicity or race are alike. Yu-fen, you are frustrated with that book and maybe felt annoyed by Eric's comment. If you were, you can tell him you don't like that.

In order to establish a context of common cultural traits and norms, Table 3.1 provides some information on values, characteristics, toys, games, as well as practice recommendations identified by Gil and Drewes (2005). This information may be helpful in selecting familiar toys for diverse children as well as identifying play themes related to diverse families. Again, each child must be uniquely understood through the RESPECTUL manner.

Table 3.1 Values and Characteristics by Prominent Diverse Groups

Diverse group	*Common values and characteristics*
African American	Interdependence and collective survival via strong kinship bonds
	Emotional vitality with vociferous expressions of feelings
	Strength and resilience through religious faith
	Parents instill pride in being Black as well as awareness of racial discrimination
	May mistrust healthcare professionals; hesitant to reveal "family business"
	Involved mother–child relationships
	Active parental monitoring and physical discipline
	Young children expected to respect elders
	Play is for young children; sports and organized activities are for older children
	Traditional gender stereotypes in children's play with boys wrestling and girls playing house (Hinds, 2005; Kotchick & Forehand, 2002)
Mexican American (Hispanic)	Male dominance and authority (Machismo)
	Interdependence over independence
	Strong extended families with communal parenting
	Value family privacy
	Catholic faith and possible reliance on Curanderos (folk healers)
	Permissive discipline of children
	Personalismo—warm personal contact first with father, mother, and then child
	"La platica"—light conversation before sensitive topics
	Varying acculturation levels within family
	Games: Juego De La Oca, Serpientes Y Escareras, & La Loteria (Hopkins, Huici, & Bermudez, 2005; Robles, 2006)

Diverse group	Common values and characteristics
Chinese American	Collectivism and importance of extended family Patriarchal family structures Unquestionable authority and parental control for children to be well-behaved, hard-working, and have academic achievement Future goal-orientation Permissive with young children, but authoritarian with older children Shame and face-saving reactions; may be hesitate to share concerns Prefer educational toys and activities Boys are encouraged to by physical and construct; girls are to be calm and nurturing Expects a directive, educational approach Reserved in expressing feelings; communicates displeasure through nonverbal cues (Kao, 2005; Kao & Landreth, 2001)
Native American	Collectivistic, cooperative, and noncompetitive characteristics Respect for elders, other people, and nature Involve extended family Harmony; order and balance Individual freedom and noninterference Permissive discipline yet may use shame as discipline Simplicity, generosity, and non-materialism Current impact of historical trauma and grief due to genocide and displacement Varying levels of acculturation and use of traditional healers Respect silences, listening, and humor Boys expected to be physical in play and girls more nurturing (Glover, 2005)
Economic poverty	Hunger, inconsistent hygiene, and limited medical care Children's anxiety and depression are higher than middle class Academic progress is hindered Social support may be hindered due to frequent moves Extensive demands on parents may limit involvement with children Parents may have lower nurturance/responsiveness with children Parents may have untreated PTSD or substance abuse issues (Nikulina, Widom, & Czaja, 2011; Schoon, Jones, Cheng, & Maughan, 2012; Slack, Holl, McDaniel, Yoo, & Bolger, 2004)
Children of gays and lesbians	Unique and innovative in family structure Greater equity in child care and household duties than heterosexual families Schools may not be open and welcoming to their families Possible separation from primary caregivers due to lack of laws for child visitation rights As opposed to popular assumption, children's sexuality is not determined by their parent's sexuality Behavioral adjustment is equivalent to peers from heterosexual families (Bishop, 2011; Dempsey, 2010; Goldberg, Smith, & Perry-Jenkins, 2012; Tan & Baggerly, 2009; Tasker & Golombok, 1997)

Note: This information does not apply to everyone within the listed group. Each individual should be uniquely considered in a RESPECTFUL manner, particularly by considering the country or state of family origin.

Strategies to obtain cultural knowledge.   Strategies for acquiring further knowledge about specific diverse cultures include: (a) reading professional literature and books about or from a particular group; (b) cultural experiences at fairs or through travel; (c) building relationships with a cultural informant; and (d) networking with diverse cultural groups. Once basic knowledge has been developed, play therapists can honor the culture by decorating waiting rooms and playrooms with pictures and games common to the culture (Robles, 2006). In addition, play therapists can express their interest in learning about clients' culture and their experience.

PLAY THERAPIST: Iftekhar, you and I are alike in many ways. We both live in Dallas, enjoy playing with toys, and like talking to your mom. We are also different in our skin color, where are families are from, and our religion. I am excited to learn more about you and your family. Maybe you can tell me something about your country of Bangladesh and your Muslim religion that I may not know.

IFTEKHAR: I like to play cricket instead of baseball. We go to Mosque on Friday afternoons, so I can't come to play with you then.

PLAY THERAPIST: You know a fun game that many others don't know! It's important to you to go to Mosque and play at other times.

Such an open invitation will allow children and parents to see a play therapist as a cultural learner. In addition, it is prudent for play therapists to verbally express their openness to be corrected if they say or do something offensive. This openness may lessen the impact of the offense.

PLAY THERAPIST: Mrs. Jesmin, since I am still learning about your family and culture, would you please tell me if I do or say something that may be impolite or offensive.

PARENT: We are observing Ramadan right now, so it is best not to offer us any snacks.

PLAY THERAPIST: Thank you for mentioning that to me so I can respect your practices.

Knowledge of group dynamics and functioning.   Knowledge of how groups are impacted by diversity among members is essential. Group dynamics including social boundaries, perceived authority, assigned roles, and tasks require careful observation when diverse children are playing (McRae & Short, 2010). For example, does a Korean American boy maintain a distant social boundary with the play therapist while a Mexican American boy stands close by the play therapist? Does a 5-year-old boy assume authority over a 5-year-old girl while they play, relegating her to the role of nurse rather than doctor? Does an 8-year-old non-Hispanic girl from an affluent family insist the task of cleaning be done by an 8-year-old girl from a Hispanic low-income family? Such group dynamics require thoughtful therapeutic responses such as the following:

PLAY THERAPIST: Chi-Sing, you are comfortable standing over there looking at the toys. Santiago, you are comfortable standing close to me. In here, you can stand and move wherever and however you choose, even if it is different.

PLAY THERAPIST: Joshua, you wanted Katelyn to play the nurse rather than the doctor. Katelyn, you can choose to be whichever you want. In here, it is important for girls and boys to decide for themselves.

PLAY THERAPIST: Caroline, you are insisting that Maxine clean up the art supplies even though you both used them. Maxine, in here you can decide if and what you want to clean up. Some kids might not think it is fair to do all the work when others also made the mess.

Group functioning, including dependency, pairing, or alliances as well as fighting or conflict, may be impacted by the diversity among members (McRae & Short, 2010). Play therapists should ponder these questions: Which children have a higher dependency on the play therapist and how does this relate to power differentials within overall society (e.g. are Haitian children more dependent than Euro-American children)? Do children of a similar ethnicity align against a child of a different ethnicity (e.g. White children pairing up and taking toys from Native American children)? When and with whom do conflicts or fights occur (e.g. is the nonverbal behavior of a boy repeatedly ignored by a girl)? Play therapists can make therapeutic responses of reflecting feelings and facilitating understanding to increase awareness of group functioning. Consider the following:

PLAY THERAPIST: Emmanuel and Johanne, you like to ask me permission before you pick up a toy, but in here you can choose to play with anything without asking permission first.

PLAY THERAPIST: Beth and Natalie, you grabbed the necklaces away from Cheyenne. Cheyenne, you looked down when they did that. Some kids may feel angry or frustrated when others take without asking. You can choose to tell them your feelings and thoughts.

PLAY THERAPIST: Sheryl, you keep talking and talking and want Mike to answer. Mike, you keep turning away like you are not hearing what she is saying. It seems you both want something different. You can ask for what you want from each other and each of you can decide if you are willing to do it.

Skills

Once play therapists have the knowledge to recognize how diversity is impacting the group, they need skills to enhance the healing power of group play therapy. Four skills that will be particularly helpful in group play therapy with diverse children are: (a) linking and joining; (b) responding to offensive comments and actions; (c) promoting cultural identity development; and (d) advocating for social justice.

Linking and joining. Linking and joining children by reflecting their common interests, abilities, or characteristics will communicate that their similarities are more important than their differences. "You both enjoy playing ball." "You each know how to make knots with a rope." "You both are 7 years old." Linking and joining decrease awkwardness and increase a sense of cohesion. When individual differences are noted, play therapists can balance the frequency of response between children to confirm each child is important no matter how different they are. "Kristen, you are showing us your dance moves. Joy, you are showing us your patience with organizing crayons. You both have strengths."

Responding to culturally offensive actions. Reality testing of cultural assumptions will occur with diverse children in the playroom. Since children convey prejudices and imitate biases in their play, play therapists must be ready to respond to offensive comments and actions that polarize group members. Consider this example between a 5-year-old White boy named Eric and a 6-year-old Black girl named Connie:

ERIC: I'm the ambulance driver. (Pushes toy ambulance across the floor.)

CONNIE: I'll be the doctor waiting at the hospital. (Rushes to grab the doctor's kit.)

ERIC: Girls can't be doctors—especially Black ones.

PLAY THERAPIST: Eric, you believe Black girls can't be doctors. Connie, you know you can decide to be and play anything you choose.

CONNIE: Yeah! I'm a smart girl. Plus, my mom is a doctor.

ERIC: Well my grandpa says girls are supposed to stay home and have babies, not be a doctor.

PLAY THERAPIST: Eric, your grandpa has one idea and Connie, your mom has a different idea. In here, you can decide the ways you want to play.

By recognizing this reality testing, the play therapist's response not only facilitated understanding of Eric's cultural and gender assumptions, but also posed new understanding by acknowledging Connie's challenge of the assumptions. Such therapeutic responses mitigate conflict and promote pro-social behavior. In group play therapy, children modify their prejudicial assumptions and offensive behavior in exchange for group acceptance (Ginott, 1961).

When children's comments or actions emotionally harm others, play therapists must protect children by setting therapeutic limits via acknowledging the feeling, communicating the limit, and targeting an alternative. Racial slurs or actions are presumed to harm others, even if the other child does not show a visible response. Consider the following interaction between Mitch, a 7-year-old Hispanic boy and Barnabus, a 7-year-old African American boy, who were close friends and were playing "gangsta."

BARNABUS: S'up boi, youz gon' hang hera or youz gonna roll wit me.

MICK: Na, I rolls wit you, Nig*a

PLAY THERAPIST: Mick, I know you are playing, but that "N" word can be hurtful to people. You can choose another word.

BARNABUS: Yeah, you ain't suppose to say that word.

MICK: O.K. Come on, hommie, let's roll!

PLAY THERAPIST: Barnabus, you helped remind him and Mick you changed it. You are both helpful friends.

Giving children credit for their willingness to change their behavior is just as important as setting the limit. The power of group play therapy is that children will increase their cultural sensitivity in exchange for group acceptance in real time. This positive cultural, visceral experience will become impeded in neuro-pathways so that automatic thoughts are more culturally sensitive (Beck, 2011).

Promoting cultural identity development.   Cultural identity development begins in childhood when patterns of thinking and evaluating self are influenced by cultural experiences and interactions (Bandura, 1977; Barbarin, 1993). Culturally responsive group play therapy can provide positive experiences that promote cultural identity development (Baggerly & Parker, 2005). For example, Baggerly and Parker (2005) described how components of an African worldview, specifically emotional vitality, interdependence, collective survival, and harmonious blending, were honored in CCPT as illustrated in the following dialogue (pp. 390–391).

EMOTIONAL VITALITY.

Darnel: We graduated from cooking class. [singing and dancing]

Play Therapist: You are proud of yourself for graduating! Doing that makes you so happy!

INTERDEPENDENCE.

Damon: Let's get the bad guy. I need the knife.

Saquan: I'll use it to get him. You get the handcuffs and we'll take him to jail.

Damon: OK. Bring him here.

Counselor: Damon, you decided to cooperate, and Saquan, you decided to play with him. You are working together.

COLLECTIVE SURVIVAL.

Damon: I'm cooking chicken wings and greens.

Jarik: I'll go to the store to get some Sprite.

Play Therapist: You are both doing your share of the work for dinner.

HARMONIOUS BLENDING.

Tyvin: This is my friend! He's dying. Call a doctor.

Keshaun: I'm the doctor. I'll give him a shot.

Tyvin: He's alive. He's back.

Play Therapist: There's hope! You were worried but worked together to make him come back.

As a result of group CCPT, these African American boys increased a sense of self-confidence and pride in their African American identity development. Furthermore, cultural identity development in children can contribute to community and academic achievement (Parham, White, & Ajamu, 2000). Therefore, play therapists need to implement the skill of researching specific cultural worldviews and honoring these worldviews via therapeutic responses in group play therapy.

Social justice advocacy skills.   Social justice is a key element of multicultural competency. "Increasing individual multicultural competence is not enough. The primary focus should be systemic change in policies and practices" (Zalaquett, Foley, Tillotson, Dinsmore, & Hof, 2008). Social justice has been defined as "valuing of fairness and equity in resources, rights, and treatment for marginalized individuals and groups who do not share power in society due to immigration, racial, ethnic, age, SES, religion, physical abilities, or sexual orientation" (Constantine, Hage, Kindaichi, & Bryant, 2007, p. 24). Green, McCollum, and Hays (2008) applied this concept to children. They stated "advocacy is an empowerment stratagem utilized to fully embrace and empathize with children whose voices are unheard by advocating for the child within social micro and macrocosms, encouraging them to become a part of their community, and subsequently increasing feelings of self-empowerment and belongingness" (p. 15).

Play therapists can implement social justice advocacy skills within group play therapy through a number of strategies. When an injustice is identified during a group play therapy session, the play therapist can reflect feelings about the injustice, encourage group members to voice their concerns to change agents, and commit to help advocate for needed resources. Consider this group play therapy dialogue between children who live in economic poverty.

SHERYL: Here is your plate of food that you have to make last until next week. [Hands other child a plate with play food.]

JUDITH: Oh, girl, you know that's right 'cause the winter holidays is next week and we ain't gonna get free breakfast and lunch at school.

PLAY THERAPIST: You both are worried about being hungry during the winter holidays. You have an important concern that you can ask your school social worker about. I can help if needed.

SHERYL: They don't listen to us kids.

JUDITH: Yea, our social worker can't do nothing.

PLAY THERAPIST: You believe there is not much hope for change. Yet, your voice and need is so important that together we can make a change. We can talk to your social worker and call the food bank together after our play time has ended.

Play therapists must be faithful in collaborating with children and their families in advocating for system changes. In this scenario, the play therapist may encourage the parent and child to call their school social worker as well as the food bank to ask for a creative solution to the hunger problem during the winter break. In addition, play therapists can facilitate a directive activity during the play session of writing a letter or sending an email asking legislators to ensure children do not experience hunger during the holidays.

Conclusion

Being a multiculturally competent group play therapist who effectively manages cultural issues entails much more than memorizing a few facts about cultures and toys. Rather, it is an ongoing life-long learning process, motivated by a deep respect for all children of all cultures. To honor cultural diversity of all children in group play therapy, play therapists must begin with self-awareness and a willingness to mitigate their own biases. Awareness of how cultural issues impact group processes will prime play therapists to respond therapeutically. Knowledge of the RESPECTFUL acronym will prevent play therapists from stereotyping children. Being diligent in implementing a variety of strategies to increase cultural knowledge will prepare play therapists to manage group dynamics and functioning with diverse children. Finally, the skills of linking and joining will create a positive social milieu so that therapeutic responses to culturally offensive actions encourage children to change. Skills of promoting cultural identity development and advocating for social justice help create a healthy environment in the playroom as well as the community at large. When play therapists increase their cultural awareness, knowledge, and skills, group play therapy will honor diverse children and help create healing communities for all cultures.

4   Ethical Considerations

The use of play as a therapeutic piece of relational connection usually brings to mind child play therapy. While this book is certainly bent in this direction, it also recognizes the great potential and impact of lifespan group play therapy. In consideration of this, we discuss both general ethics and ethics related to minor clients.

Readers should first be reminded to be familiar with federal, state, and local statutes governing their practice. Case law and administrative rules also come into play. Many states require that mental health licensees receive several hours of legal and ethical continuing education prior to license renewal.

Generally, ethical considerations for group play therapists are not based upon the modality of group play therapy or the theoretical approach, but rather on the ethical guidelines of licensure and professional organizations to which the therapist belongs. The licensed psychologist or professional counselors, for example, are expected to follow the standards of their respective state boards of licensure as well as the American Psychological Association and American Counseling Association if they are members.

Competence

An examination of ethics within the context of play therapy, perhaps more so group play therapy, should begin with a consideration of *competence*. Hearkening back to the definition of group play therapy in Chapter 1, it is an intervention used by "a therapist *trained* in both play therapy and group therapy procedures." Too often, health and mental health practitioners attend a brief workshop on a topic of interest and immediately adopt the practice, without obtaining needed further training and adequate supervised experience. This is an issue of competence. It is our responsibility that we always work within the scope of our expertise.

It is both clinically and ethically imperative that play therapists have adequate training and supervised experience in the field. It is an ethical mandate of all ethical codes of mental health organizations (e.g., APA, ACA, AAMFT, NASW) that clinicians practice only within the boundaries of their competence. While competence may be challenging to assess, and certainly subject to opinion, it is nevertheless an obligation for those working with any specific intervention, such as group play therapy, to have adequate training and appropriately supervised clinical experience.

The Association for Play Therapy (APT) has established a process for becoming a Registered Play Therapist (RPT) and a Registered Play Therapist-Supervisor (RPT-S). Although this is not licensure or certification, the "credential" of being a RPT or RPT-S does serve as evidence that a play therapist has met minimal training and supervised experience standards. The APT speaks on the issue of competence in their statement on *Play Therapy Best Practices* (2009):

> Play therapists practice only within the boundaries of their competence. Competence is based on training; supervised experience; state, national, and international professional credentials, and professional experience. Play therapists commit to knowledge acquisition and skill development pertinent to working with a diverse client population … Play therapists practice a new specialty after appropriate education, training, and supervised experience. Play therapists take steps to ensure the competence of their work while developing skills in the new specialty.
>
> (p. 10)

This is echoed in the *Best Practice Guidelines* of the Association for Specialists in Group Work (ASGW), as stated by Thomas and Pender (2008):

> Group Workers have a basic knowledge of groups and the principles of group dynamics, and are able to perform the core group competencies … They gain knowledge, personal awareness, sensitivity, and skills pertinent to working with a diverse client population. Additionally, Group Workers have adequate understanding and skill in any group specialty area chosen for practice (psychotherapy, counseling, task, psychoeducation, as described in the ASGW Training Standards).
>
> (p. 115)

A specific example of the aspiration for clinical expertise in working with play therapy and group play therapy is the respect for developmental capabilities. A group play therapy intervention that is superb for adults may or may not be developmentally appropriate for children—and vice versa. Honoring developmental differences, while avoiding unneeded rigidity, is a reflection of competence.

The second issue related to competence is the legal status of minors in a given municipality. Fundamentally, minors are considered legally incompetent, until an established age as decided by the state. The presumption of the state is that minors are legally incompetent. This means that children are not considered to have the legal capacity to consent (or refuse) services, or the right to obtain and retain privilege in regards to confidential information. It is the legal guardian, which is most often the parent, who is the holder of these rights. This can make the legal and ethical aspect of counseling children occasionally ambiguous for all involved persons.

The focus of treatment in child play therapy is generally upon the child; however, the exclusion of the parents from the process is both impractical and unethical. In most cases, the parents are not only the significant caretakers, they are also the ones who are legally responsible for the child.

There are particular considerations in providing mental health treatment to children. Therapists need to consider a variety of questions, including the following summary (Corey, Corey, & Callanan, 2007):

- Can minors consent to treatment without parental knowledge and parental consent?
- At what age can a minor consent to treatment?
- To what degree should minors be allowed to participate in setting the goals of therapy and in providing consent to undergo it?
- What are the limits of confidentiality in counseling minors? Would you discuss these limits with minor clients even though a parent or guardian consents to treatment of the minor?
- What does informed consent consist of when working with minors?

(p. 187)

Confidentiality and Children

In most circumstances, parental consent is needed to authorize treatment for children. Thus, parents have the right to information about their child's treatment. As a result, confidentiality generally cannot be fully promised to a minor. This may present a challenge to therapists looking to establish a therapeutic relationship. Play therapists cannot promise their clients that everything shared, whether verbally or nonverbally, will not be shared with the parents. This dilemma will be further discussed below, following some general comments about confidentiality.

There is frequently some level of confusion among therapists concerning the differences between the terms *privacy, confidentiality,* and *privilege.* Fundamentally, privacy basically means that people have the right to choose what others may or may not know about them; confidentiality refers to the codified ethical responsibility of the therapist to respect and therefore limit access to the personal information of clients; and privilege refers to the legal responsibility of therapists to protect client confidentiality (Sweeney, 2001). Essentially, confidentiality is an ethical obligation that the therapist owes to the client (confidentiality therefore is *owned* by the client), and privileged communication is a legal concept that protects the rights of clients from having information disclosed.

For minors, the guardian, most often the parent, is the legal authority and decision maker. Only the guardian or parent can authorize treatment and can obtain information about the therapeutic process (including diagnosis, treatment plan, etc.). This legal authority may be restricted to the person with legal and/or physical custody, or the minor if emancipated or authorized by law to receive treatment. This varies according to state law. Any therapist who works with children should be aware of state and local statutes regarding parental rights.

All therapists should be aware of the basic exceptions to confidentiality. Although these may vary slightly from state to state, these exceptions include the following: disclosure of child or elder abuse; disclosure of an intent to commit harm to self or others; written authorization by the parent or guardian; a legal action brought against the therapist which is initiated by the client; and when ordered by a court to release information (Sweeney, 2001). It is imperative that play therapists are aware of the mandated reporting laws in the state in which they practice, as well as other case and statute law which affect confidentiality in the therapy process. When it is necessary and appropriate to release confidential information, therapists should disclose the minimal amount of confidential material needed in order to comply with the specific situation.

Confidentiality and Group Therapy

The ethical responsibility to maintain confidentiality obviously extends to group therapy. However, therapists cannot guarantee that group members will guarantee the confidence and privacy of other group members. The importance of maintaining confidentiality should be communicated to the group, but therapists can only guarantee their own maintenance of confidentiality and privilege. Remley and Herlihy (2005) emphasize: "Despite the fact that others in the room might not keep a client's secrets, a counselor's responsibility is not diminished by the presence of additional persons in a counseling session" (p. 113).

It is the group therapist's responsibility to communicate this dynamic to group members, emphasizing the importance of confidentiality while not being able to unconditionally guarantee it for and by other group members. Thomas and Pender (2008), in the *Best Practice Guidelines* of the ASGW, state:

> Group Workers define confidentiality and its limits (for example, legal and ethical exceptions and expectations; waivers implicit with treatment plans, documentation and insurance usage). Group Workers have the responsibility to inform all group participants of the need for confidentiality, potential consequences of breaching confidentiality and that legal privilege does not apply to group discussions (unless provided by state statute).
>
> (p. 114)

Although group members who violate other group members' confidentiality generally do not face legal consequences (Lasky & Riva, 2006), not only are group leaders bound to confidentiality and privilege, they should teach the group of its importance to the group. This should also be part of the informed consent documentation which clients sign prior to the therapy process.

Informed Consent

Based upon the general ethical principles of autonomy and respect, all clients in individual and group psychotherapy have the right and authority to consent to services. All persons who enter into therapy have the fundamental right to make decisions that affect their well-being, and therefore need to consider the potential benefits and risks of these decisions. With regard to any counseling intervention (including group play therapy), informed consent refers to the decision of clients whether to engage in treatment, what happens during the course of treatment, and what information the therapist may disclose to third parties (Sales, DeKraai, Hall, & Duvall, 2008).

There are several elements of the informed consent process (Sweeney, 2001). One is that the therapist must disclose all relevant information about the process to the client. This involves more than the basic discussion of office policies. This may be especially important for the group play therapist, as the rationale for and the process of play therapy and group play therapy is often unclear to people—particularly children and parents. Another component of informed consent is the client's comprehension of this information. This must be followed by a voluntary agreement to participate in therapy, free from undue influence or coercion. These will be commented upon further below.

To further detail the principle of informed consent, the consent of clients must be given in a voluntary, knowledgeable, and competent state. For child clients, this is where the issue becomes somewhat complex. Because of their legal status as minors, children are generally not considered voluntary, knowledgeable, and competent clients. Play therapists choose to use play as a means of connecting and communicating with children because they lack the developmental skills to engage in therapy in the same manner as adult clients. Informed consent is a sophisticated and abstract concept and therefore counter to this basic rationale for using play therapy. Nevertheless, informed consent remains an ethical and therapeutic imperative.

Since children are generally considered legally incapable of consenting to the process of play therapy, a substitute must make the decision (Sweeney, 2001): "In most cases, this will be the parent or legal guardian. In cases where the parent is not involved, the therapist must ensure that the person providing the consent is legally able to do so. A grandparent or other relative, who is not the legal guardian, generally cannot provide consent" (p. 68). When working with a child case involving a divorce situation, it is important that therapists be aware of the state laws concerning custody and parental rights. Some states permit both the primary and non-primary custodian to consent for treatment (and to review records), while others do not.

Additionally, there are exceptions to the general requirement for the legal guardian's consent to treatment, which also vary from state to state. Some examples include emergency treatment situations; the case of an emancipated minor; drug and alcohol treatment for children (generally aged 12 or older); counseling for birth control, pregnancy, or sexually transmitted diseases; and other specific situations as outlined by statute (Sweeney, 2001).

It is also important to note that informed consent is not a one-time event at the beginning of the therapeutic process. This may be particularly important for the play and expressive therapist to know. Since group play therapy may involve a variety of creative and projective activities throughout the course of the group process, it is important to receive consent for any new activity. This obviously includes the freedom to opt out of an activity at the beginning or during the course of the process, as we know that expressive activities can be quite emotionally evocative and provocative.

Professional Disclosure

It is the group play therapist's responsibility to provide information about their professional identity and office policies to clients, parents, and children when developmentally appropriate. This "professional disclosure statement," which is required by law in some states, should educate the client about several items, including such specifics as:

(1) information about the orientation of the group play therapist in regards to theory and technique; (2) degrees and credential held by the therapist; (3) specific training and supervised experience relevant to the therapist's practice; (4) information about fee schedules and payment process; (5) limits to confidentiality; (6) process of working with insurance companies; and (7) other information pieces specific to a therapist's practice which ensure that the client is fully aware of the process and therapist's qualifications to be involved in that process (Sweeney, 2001).

Erford (2011) outlines specific items that should be included in the professional disclosure statements for group play therapists:

- The professional preparation of the group worker (e.g., education; training; licenses held, with the addresses of the licensing boards; certifications held, with the addresses of the certifying bodies; theoretical orientation).
- The nature of the group services provided (e.g., the nature, purpose[s], and goals of the group).
- The role and responsibility of group leaders and group members, including expectations for member behavior in the group.
- The limits and exceptions to confidentiality with regard to group member health information and disclosures made during the group, especially with regard to individuals coerced into group attendance by third parties.
- Policies regarding psychoactive substance.
- Policies regarding contact or personal involvement among group members outside the group.
- Policies regarding attendance at group meetings and procedures to be followed in the event of absences.
- Documentation requirements and required disclosure of information to others.
- Procedures for consultation between (among) group leader(s) and group member(s).
- Fees and billing information.
- Time parameters of the group.
- Potential effects of group participation.

(p. 27)

It is recommended to discuss both professional disclosure and informed consent with children and adolescents, even if they are not the legal holders of consent and disclosure. In a developmentally appropriate manner, it is an empowering process to include them in this process. While children and adolescents may not be holders of privilege, they are nevertheless entitled to confidentiality, and they have the right to know about their counselor's credentials and policies. This will serve as a further means to beginning and developing the therapeutic relationship.

Children and Parental Rights

Since children are the frequent recipients of group play therapy services, it is helpful to consider the legal and ethical rights that both parties have. Remembering that there is some degree of variance from state to state, the following rights are summarized by Prout and Prout (2007):

- Children in therapy have the right:
  - To be informed about the evaluation process and reasons and results in understandable terms.
  - To be informed about therapeutic interventions and rationale in understandable terms.
  - To be informed about confidentiality and its limitations.
  - To control release of information.
  - Not to be involved in therapy if uncomfortable or unsuccessful (this is not always possible when it is mandated by court order or IEP).
  - To be treated with respect and told the truth.
  - To participate with the therapist and/or parent(s) in decision making and goal setting.
  - Not to be labeled the scapegoat in a dysfunctional family.
- Parents' right and responsibilities include the:
  - Legal responsibility to provide for their child's welfare.
  - Right to access to information (educational, medical, therapeutic) that pertains to their child's welfare.
  - Right to seek therapy and/or treatment services for their child.
  - Right to be involved in therapeutic decision making and goal setting for their child.
  - Right to give permission for treatments.
  - Right to release confidential information concerning their child.

(pp. 41–42)

A few things come to mind when considering this list. It is the group play therapist's responsibility to understand ethics and law, deliver information and written material in a developmentally appropriate manner, and balance the rights of children and parents. The best interests of the clients have to be of utmost concern, regardless of age.

Records in Group Work

The group play therapist has the responsibility to maintain records that are professionally adequate, appropriately secure, and retained for a prescribed length of time (Sweeney, 2001). While it may be generally acknowledged that many persons in the helping professions do not care for the administrative aspect of their job, it is nevertheless a crucial and required necessity.

All therapists are responsible for the production and maintenance of records. These include, but would not be limited to: intake information, basic office forms (informed consent, office policies [billing information, cancellation fee policy, etc.], professional disclosure statements, release forms, etc.), client history, psychological tests, progress notes, treatment plans, etc. A reasonable standard for play therapists to consider in the maintenance of a client file would be if they would feel comfortable having the file sub-poenaed and reviewed by a court and professional peers (Sweeney, 2001).

Record-keeping for group therapy brings up some unique questions and challenges. It is a decision for the group play therapist whether to maintain one file for all group members, or separate files for group members. Christner, Stewart, and Freeman (2007) summarize this challenge:

> If records are kept for the group as a whole, which may correspond more closely to the way the therapist experiences and thinks about the group session, it creates a problem of confidentiality with regard to access to records by group members, release of the record to third parties, and subpoenas of the entire record if a court proceeding involves one of the group members. However, if records are kept for each individual group member, it may be difficult to capture the context of a group member's comments, and how he or she related to the other group members. The challenge is to maintain the confidentiality of group members while still being able to follow the flow of the session. This makes record keeping more complex for group therapists than for individual therapists.
>
> (p. 81)

Some group therapists maintain notes about group members in individual files, avoiding specific or identifying references to other group members. For the sake of maintaining appropriate confidentiality and privilege, this is the safest policy, while recognizing this does create more work for the group therapist. Some therapists additionally maintain a group file, in order to keep track of the flow of the group therapy process, as well as interventions used. There is simply no way of predicting who will want access to the records.

We recommend the maintenance of individual files for each group member. The group play therapists can then use a generic form that includes what has generally occurred in the group play therapy process, which can then be photocopied for each individual file, with additional individual notes being added for each member. While it does take practice and skill (and additional time) to write out individual notes, it does assure confidentiality for each group member.

Records should be secured appropriately. It is recommended that client files be stored in a locked file cabinet, behind two locked doors (the office door, and the door to the room where the records are stored). If using computer records, they should be encrypted and properly secured.

Concerning the appropriate length of time for which to keep client records, most states and professional organizations have stated minimums. Therapists should be well acquainted with these laws in the state in which they practice. Since play therapy is frequently done with children, it is recommended that records for child clients are stored for the corresponding number of years beyond the age of majority. While the storing of records may be cumbersome, particularly in terms of space, it is always better to store records for too long than not long enough (Sweeney, 2001).

Additionally, therapists are responsible for ensuring that all persons having access to files, such as support staff, are trained in the appropriate and confidential handling of client records. Therapists are liable for errors (mistaken or purposeful) made by persons in their employ.

The Use of Techniques

We support the use of a wide variety of techniques in the process of group play therapy. This is evidenced in many chapters of this book. In the preface, we propose some basic questions to consider in the use of techniques: (a) Is the technique developmentally appropriate? (b) What theory underlies the technique? and (c) What is the therapeutic intent in employing a given technique? (Sweeney, 2011). These are proposed as clinically significant considerations. They are also ethically imperative questions as well.

Corey et al. (2011) discuss how group techniques can be abused or used unethically. These include group therapists using techniques: (1) with which they are unfamiliar; (2) to enhance their power; (3) whose purpose is to create intensity because of the therapist's need for intensity; and (4) to pressure members who have expressed a desire not to participate in an exercise.

A set of guidelines is proposed by Corey et al. (2011) regarding the use of techniques in the group therapy process, all of which arguably apply to group play therapy:

- Techniques used have a therapeutic purpose and are grounded in some theoretical framework.
- The client's self-exploration and self-understanding is fostered.
- Techniques are devised for the unique needs of various cultural and ethnic groups.
- Techniques are modified so that they are suitable for the client's cultural and ethnic background.
- Techniques are used to enhance the group process rather than to cover up the leader's incompetence.
- Techniques are introduced in a timely and sensitive manner and are abandoned if they are not working.
- The tone of a leader is consistently invitational; members are given the freedom either to participate in or to skip a given experiment.
- Leaders use techniques in which they have received training and supervision.

(p. 501)

Our perspective is that group play therapists should not be afraid to use techniques, but should be appropriately trained and supervised—and should know about both the benefits and the potential detriment of techniques. While it is not possible to know about all possible responses to a specific technique or intervention, group play therapists should know how to address both expected and unexpected outcomes.

Emotional release and catharsis may be the intent or perhaps an unexpected outcome of a given group play therapy technique. There may be a delayed or immediate need to address a group member's response to a given technique. If there is considerable distress, therapists have the clinical and ethical responsibility to address this. Thus, while the use of time in the group play therapy process is often seen as primarily a clinical issue, it may become an ethical issue in light of a client's negative response to the use of a given intervention.

   It has already been recommended that group play therapists receive adequate training and supervised experience. It may also be appropriate for us to experience being a member of a group and participating in group play therapy interventions prior to using them in the role of a therapist. We can learn the emotional and behavioral power of a given technique, and the potential stress that may eventuate. If we are going to model respect as a therapist, we need to have appropriate knowledge and respect for the techniques we employ.

Screening and Selection of Group Members

Screening of potential group members is discussed in Chapter 5. It should be additionally noted that this is an ethical issue as well as a clinical one. The ASGW states that: "Group Workers screen prospective group members if appropriate to the type of group being offered. When selection of group members is appropriate, Group Workers identify group members whose needs and goals are compatible with the goals of the group" (Thomas & Pender, 2008, p. 114). Corey et al. (2011) suggest a pertinent question in this regard: "Is it appropriate for *this* person to become a participant in *this* type of group, with *this* leader, at *this* time?" (p. 491).

   While screening may be a personal or theoretical issue for a given therapist, we would argue that it is always appropriate to do some type of screening prior to a person joining a therapeutic play group. This becomes an issue of client welfare—not just for an individual in the group, but also for the group as a whole. We have to consider, as part of the screening process, whether the presence of any given group member is in the best interests of other group members.

Referrals

There are several circumstances in which the therapist must make a referral. This is an important issue to consider from an ethical perspective. The group play therapist must always keep the best interests of the group member in mind, and the situation may call for a referral for different or adjunct services.

   When there is reasonable evidence that a group member's situation requires medical evaluation, the therapist must make a referral to a physician. Even if it is the judgment of the therapist that a symptom is most likely psychosomatic in origin, a referral for medical evaluation is nevertheless the appropriate course of action. If there is a need for psychiatric evaluation and medication, the referral must be made.

   When and if it becomes evident that a group member requires additional care, there needs to be a referral for individual therapy or some other type of adjunct services. A question that has not yet been discussed in this chapter is whether or not the provider of individual services should be provided by the same group play therapist or another provider.

   While it cannot be argued that it is unethical for a therapist to concurrently provide individual and group therapy services for the same client, it will frequently be an awkward and delicate clinical situation. If a group play therapist has a simultaneous therapeutic relationship with one (or several) group members, it may be difficult to separate the two relationships—for the therapist and the client. It may also make other group members who do not have an individual therapeutic relationship with the group therapist jealous. We would advise against this dynamic, but recognize that this will be variable based on several dynamics.

Additionally, group play therapists should be cautioned against doing individual therapy within the group context. If a group member needs additional consultation or clinical attention, this should be done outside of the group's established clinical time, recognizing boundaries for both the therapist and client.

The awareness of clinical competence has been discussed above. When a client situation is beyond the group play therapist's scope of expertise, it is clearly necessary to make an appropriate referral. The group play therapist has a legal and ethical responsibility to make the referral to an appropriately competent clinician, and must make the referral and transfer of the client in a competent fashion. It is possible that there would be legal liability for the referring therapist if the referral source acts in a negligent or incompetent manner (Sweeney, 2001).

Conclusion

There are several guidelines that are always helpful when dealing with legal and ethical issues. It is always helpful and frequently necessary to consult with other professionals in the field. Ongoing supervision is clearly helpful in terms of professional growth as a clinician, but also as a resource concerning ethical matters. Honest and open dialog with clients is also an imperative from a legal and ethical perspective (Sweeney, 2001). Clients are always more likely to file a complaint or legal action against a professional when they feel ignored and discounted—empathy always matters! Finally, all legal or ethical concerns should be carefully documented in the client record.

Therapists who work with clients using the modality of group play therapy do so because of a commitment to reaching clients through this unique expressive and projective medium of communication. This process may not be well understood by children, adolescents, adults, and other therapists and the general public. It is important that group play therapists educate the wider field of mental health and the general public about the process and benefits of play therapy in the context of group counseling.

5 Group Play Therapy Procedures and Stages

There are basic group play therapy procedures that cross both theoretical and technical considerations. These include the process of selecting group members, group size, balancing group members, group play therapy room and materials, length and frequency of sessions, necessary group play therapy skills, group phases/stages, and assessing progress and readiness for termination. While theoretical orientation and specific techniques may change, these elements are crucial to understand and implement.

Selection of Group Members

The selection of group members in group play therapy is as important as in any therapeutic group. Yalom (2005) suggests that group therapy members may end up being discouraged and may not receive help if careful selection is not employed. It is both a clinical and ethical responsibility. In regard to screening of group members, the Association for Play Therapy (2009) notes: "The play therapist selects clients for group play therapy whose needs are compatible and conducive to the therapeutic process and well-being of each client" (p. 6).

Erford (2011) poses important questions for screening and selecting group members, which apply to group play therapy as well as any therapeutic group:

- What are the potential member needs? Does the applicant need the sort of intervention or experience offered in the planned group?
- What are the applicant's abilities? Does the applicant have the prerequisite knowledge, skills, and attitudes necessary to succeed at the sort of personal and interpersonal challenges that will be posed during the group?
- What are the applicant's personal and interpersonal limitations? Does the applicant have personal or interpersonal qualities that would make success in the group difficult or impossible or that would seriously interfere with others' success?

(p. 80)

Ginott (1975) asserts that the basic requirement for selection to a play therapy group is the presence of and capacity for "social hunger." This basically refers to children's need to be accepted by their peers and a desire to attain and maintain status in the group. Consistent with this, Yalom (2005) contends that any client's motivation to participate and work is the key variable for selection and inclusion. Both Ginott's and Yalom's perspectives arguably apply to potential group members of all ages.

Selection for and participation in group play therapy is obviously a case-by-case clinical decision. Ginott (1961) suggests several contraindications:

- Siblings who exhibit intense rivalry.
- Extremely aggressive children.
- Sexually acting-out children.
- Children experiencing difficulty due to poor infant–mother attachment.
- Sociopathic children (intending to inflict harm or revenge).
- Children with an extremely poor self-image.

We would contend, however, that these suggested contraindications might be debatable. Under the appropriate therapeutic conditions, these children may well benefit from the group play therapy experience. Ginott's purpose may be surmised as intending to protect children and therapists. Appropriate training and supervised experience, however, can mitigate these safety concerns.

Naturally, interviewing potential group play therapy members is imperative. For children, this will involve meeting with parents. For potential child group members, using individual play therapy as part of the process of screening for potential group play therapy members is generally recommended. Even a single play session may reveal the indication or contraindication for inclusion in a group. This may also be helpful for adolescents and adults. For example, prior to including adolescents or adults in group sandtray therapy, it may be helpful to do individual sandtrays for screening purposes.

Other screening methods may be appropriate, including parent and/or teacher report, behavioral or other formal assessment, child interviews, group interviews, and other historical resources.

Obviously, not all people are appropriate for group play therapy. These may include people who are overly aggressive or dominating, hypersensitive to criticism, narcissistic, and extremely anxious or depressed. Generally, people with severe psychopathology may not be appropriate for group play therapy, and may need individual work prior to or instead of group participation.

Also, it should be noted that some clients (of all ages) simply do not respond well to group play therapy. These clients can be seen on an individual play therapy basis, or they may be candidates for filial or family play therapy. Several issues may be considered in these cases—the client is simply not ready for a group experience, the presenting problem may lend itself to another intervention, or group work may be contraindicated for psychological or physiological safety concerns.

Group Size and Balance

There are many considerations in regard the appropriate size for play therapy groups. First, it is important to note that a therapeutic group can reasonably be defined as consisting of two or more unrelated clients. While this is an obvious point, it underscores that there is not a minimal group size. This does lead us to a second crucial point, regarding the reasonable maximum number of group members. All therapeutic groups should have a maximum number of clients based on the therapist's ability to appropriately attend and facilitate therapeutic dynamics.

This maximum is too often ignored. The therapeutic value of play therapy groups can easily be compromised by the ignorant attempt to have too many group members. This is a clinical decision, which should be determined by both counseling theory and planned interventions, rather than factors of expediency or administrative issues.

O'Connor (2000) suggests the following criteria in determining the makeup of a play therapy group:

1. There should be no more than four to six children in a group run by one adult, and no more than six to ten children in a group with two adults.
2. There should be no more than a 3-year age spread among the group members, especially among younger children.
3. The socioeconomic status and/or the children's ethnic background should be somewhat similar. This may be one of the least important variables unless the differences between the children are very dramatic, in which case the group may become focused on these issues and unable to address other content or behavioral areas.
4. The children should all be within 15 IQ points of one another.
5. The ability to mix boys and girls within a group varies with the age of the children, the type of group, and the goals of the intervention. There is no fixed rule, but is a dimension you should consider.

(p. 417)

These suggestions provide a springboard upon which to discuss several variables regarding group selection and makeup.

We would suggest that four to six children would be an absolute maximum for child group play therapy, and may be too large. It can be quite challenging to adequately therapeutically attend to six children, in light of the considerable activity level. This may be mitigated by the level of structure and prescribed activity that may be involved. With adolescents and adults, it is often easier to have slightly larger numbers in a therapeutic play group. We would suggest that the younger the group members, the smaller the group.

The decision to do co-therapy in group play therapy may again be related to the structure and intent of the therapeutic play group. We would suggest that this be related to the size of the group, the developmental level of group members, and the size of the group facility (and its corresponding ability to handle the number of people in the room).

In terms of the age spread, we would suggest for children that the age range not exceed 12 months. Note that we have *not* said 1 year. The difference between a 4-year-old and a 5-year-old can be substantial—especially if we are talking about a child who has just turned 4 and a child who is about to turn 6. The developmental differences are substantial. This brings up an important issue—it is crucial to consider developmental age more so than chronological age. Age spread becomes less important with adolescents and adults, and is generally not an issue when doing sibling group play therapy.

O'Connor's (2000) comments on socioeconomic status and/or ethnicity may or may not be important and applicable. As he notes, it is essentially a clinical decision. This also applies to his suggestion about an IQ range of 15 points. We would suggest that it is generally not necessary to assess for intelligence or aptitude, unless there is a compelling related issue that affects ability to socially interact.

In regard to mixing gender, this more often applies to children, where we would generally suggest that there is no need to separate based on gender until middle school or junior high school. Also, depending on group topic, there is no need to separate based on gender for adolescent and adult therapeutic play groups. This will again be a clinical decision.

Another variable to consider for child play therapy groups may be the physical size of children. For example, in a small group of two or three children, mixing inordinately small or large children may create an uncomfortable, awkward, or inappropriate dynamic.

There are other issues of balance to consider. It may be helpful to balance group members between relatively equal numbers of shy and withdrawn children with outgoing and assertive children. There can be benefit for both populations. Sweeney (2011a) also suggests: "Whereas it is often helpful to run groups on particular topics and for particular populations, it may be appropriate to avoid composing a group of children who have experienced the same trauma to prevent an escalation of traumatic behaviors or emotions. This should be the judgment call of the play therapist" (p. 233).

Therapy Room and Materials

Group play therapy should be conducted in a facility of adequate size and with appropriate materials. Sweeney (2011a) and Sweeney and Homeyer (1999) emphasize that a regular counseling office may not be appropriate, because of the need to set too many limits. A therapy room that includes typical office equipment will often necessitate setting limits in order to protect the office and its contents. This increased need for limits can create a restrictive environment, reducing the permissive atmosphere that is so helpful in the group play therapy process.

It is not unusual for group therapy rooms to be equipped with carpeting, multiple chairs, and soft pillows. The group play therapy room, particularly for younger children, may well have different needs.

A group play therapy room that is set aside for therapeutic play groups is ideal. This may or may not be possible in some therapeutic settings. A group play therapy room that is floored with tile and equipped with sturdy furniture and toys is preferable. An adequately sized room is important. Sweeney (2011a) notes:

> The room should obviously not be too small or too large—at least 12 by 15 feet is suggested. A playroom that is too small can lead to frustration and aggression among group members. The room that is too large not only creates the possibility of uncontrolled behavior but also enables the withdrawn child to avoid interaction.

Because there is considerable potential for high levels of noise and messiness, the location of the group room in a counseling facility is an important consideration.

(p. 234)

The location of a group play therapy room in an agency or other setting is often an important consideration. Play therapy with an individual client is often a noisy process. Naturally, the group play therapy process often multiplies this, and may cause some level of disturbance. A location that will in some way limit this disturbance is preferable.

The group play therapy materials will often vary according to theoretical orientation or specific therapeutic intent. Landreth (2012) suggests general characteristics of toys and materials in play therapy that are considered cross-theoretical and applicable to most group play therapy situations. Materials should:

1. Facilitate a wide range of creative expression.
2. Facilitate a wide range of emotional expression.
3. Engage children's interests.
4. Facilitate expressive and exploratory play.
5. Allow exploration and expression without verbalization.
6. Allow success without prescribed structure.
7. Allow for noncommittal play.
8. Have sturdy construction for active use.

(p. 156)

Landreth (2012) also notes that play materials should be carefully selected, as opposed to being generally collected. This should again be related to theoretical approach and/or therapeutic intent. Nash and Schaefer (2011) echo this: "The selection of toys and other items to be included certainly varies, depending on the therapist's theoretical orientation, personal ideas and values, and budget/space issues ... a general rule is that every item in the playroom should serve a therapeutic purpose" (p. 7).

Another consideration is that it may *not* be appropriate to provide enough toys or play materials of any one type so that each group member can have one. Whereas this may seem to promote fairness, group play therapy clients can lose the opportunity to learn to share and resolve conflict with limited group play therapy materials.

Length and Frequency of Sessions

It is important to consider the length of each group play therapy session. We would suggest a recommended guideline to relate the length of the group session to the age of the members. When working with children, the younger the child group members are, generally, the shorter the session. The therapeutic play group facilitator should always consider the attention span of the children, again considering developmental age over chronological age. For preschool children and early elementary-age children, a play therapy group may run for 20 to 40 minutes. For preadolescent children approaching middle or junior high school, the group may run well over an hour.

A consideration that is not often discussed is the stamina of the group play therapist. If there are several children in the group and the therapist is actively participating and communicating empathy and acceptance to *all* group members, the process may simply be more tiring than adult group play therapy. Fundamentally, a fatigued therapist will find it challenging to be an empathic one.

The duration of the group process will also vary. This may depend on play therapy groups meeting in different settings (schools, hospitals, etc.) and with different populations (sexually abused, grieving, etc.).

The frequency of therapeutic play groups may correspond with the purpose of the group, the clinical setting, and the severity of the presenting problem. Intensive short-term groups, meeting two to five times per week—if logistically possible—may be very effective. Tyndall-Lind, Landreth, and Giordano (2001) reported the significant efficacy of intensive group play therapy with children who have witnessed domestic violence, noting reductions in problem behaviors, depression, and anxiety, as well as increases in self-esteem.

Group Play Therapy Skills

The group play therapist's skills begin with the skills needed for a group therapist in general. Although not specific to group play therapy, according to the Association for Specialists in Group Work (2000), the following skills are needed for group leaders:

- collaborative consultation with targeted populations to enhance ecological validity of planned group interventions
- planning for a group work activity including such aspects as developing overarching purpose, establishing goals and objectives, detailing methods to be used in achieving goals and objectives, determining methods for outcome assessment, and verifying ecological validity of plan
- encouraging participation of group members
- attending to, describing, acknowledging, confronting, understanding, and responding empathically to group member behavior
- attending to, acknowledging, clarifying, summarizing, confronting, and responding empathically to group member statements
- attending to, acknowledging, clarifying, summarizing, confronting, and responding empathically to group themes
- eliciting information from and imparting information to group members
- providing appropriate self-disclosure
- maintaining group focus; keeping a group on task
- giving and receiving feedback in a group setting
- contributing to evaluation activities during group participation
- engaging in self-evaluation of personally selected performance goals
- evidencing ethical practice in planning, observing, and participating in group activities
- evidencing best practice in planning, observing, and participating in group activities

- evidencing diversity-competent practice in planning, observing, and participating in group activities.

(pp. 6–8)

This is consistent with those skills suggested and encouraged by several authors on group counseling and therapy, including Corey (2012), Gladding (2012), Yalom and Leszcz (2005), and Jacobs, Masson, Harvill, and Schimmel (2012).

We would assert that an overriding skill, or perhaps a group leading principle, is the ability to facilitate. Directing a group may be called for, but facilitating the group process tends to have greater therapeutic impact. This again can be viewed within a cross-theoretical context. Group facilitation involves a sensitivity to group members' emotional and relational needs, and is reflected by the facilitator's assistance in establishing a sense of belonging and esteem among group members. Group members value the process and value themselves when they feel respect, belonging, investment, and responsibility—all of which are developed when the group leader establishes a culture of facilitation and inclusion.

Punctuating this dynamic, Sweeney (2011a) notes:

> The primary role of the group play therapist is to remain a facilitator of the process. … While change is dependent on group members, it is important to remember that the therapist's role continues to include aspects such as the instillation of hope, promotion of altruism and universality, development of social skills, and promotion of imitative behavior and catharsis.

(p. 236)

Group play therapists should have adequate training and supervised experience in both play therapy and group therapy, prior to combining the two. Group play therapy is an advanced play therapy skill. Ray (2011) reminds us that "group play therapy demands not only the expertise of the therapist in play therapy, but also an expertise in facilitation" (p. 183) with more than one child in the process.

Finally, we would agree with Landreth's (2012) suggestions for the needed personality characteristics for play therapists in general. In light of the inherent increase in process and activity level between individual and group play therapy, these characteristics are all the more important when working with more than one play therapy client:

- Objective and flexible
- Does not judge or evaluate
- Open-minded
- Patient
- High tolerance for ambiguity
- Future-minded
- Personal courage
- Being real, warmth and caring, acceptance, and sensitive understanding
- Personally secure
- Sense of humor.

(pp. 99–103)

Group Phases/Stages

Group play therapy may or may not be phase- or stage-oriented. This can depend on the therapist's theoretical orientation, the therapeutic structure of the group process, or administrative format of the group. Before discussion of play therapy group stages, it is helpful to look at group therapy stages in general.

Bergin and Klein (2009) suggest four basic stages that most groups proceed through: initial, transition, working, and termination. They emphasize that movement from stage to stage is rarely smooth and uniform.

Corey (2012) expands on this, and talks about six stages. The first stage involves *Pregroup Issues*, focused on the formation of the group—which includes announcing the group, recruiting members, screening/selecting group members, and determining group functioning. The second stage is the *Initial Stage*, focused on orientation and exploration—which includes determination of group structure, group members getting acquainted, and exploration of group members' expectations. The third stage is the *Transition Stage*, focused on dealing with issues of resistance and ambivalence among group members—which includes issues of anxiety, defensiveness, and the struggle for control. The fourth stage is called the *Working Stage*, focused on group cohesion and productivity—which includes increased group cohesion and trust, leading to greater communication and mutual feedback. The fifth stage is the *Final Stage*, focused on consolidation and termination—which includes group members applying lessons learned in group, discovering meaning from the group process, and moving towards summarization and termination. Finally, in the sixth stage, there are *Postgroup Issues*, focused on evaluation of the group process and follow-up—which includes evaluating the group outcome, and the suggestion for a follow-up group session to discuss the group experience as well as perspective for group members.

Yalom and Leszcz (2005) discuss "formative stages of the group" (p. 309). In the *Initial Stage*, there are issues of orientation, hesitant participation, search for meaning, and dependency (p. 311). In the *Second Stage*, the issues include conflict, dominance, and rebellion (p. 314). In the *Third Stage*, there is a development of cohesion (p. 319). More important than these "stages," perhaps, Yalom and Leszcz discuss key therapeutic factors in group therapy that do not necessarily develop in a stage/phase fashion. These include:

- *Instillation of hope*—group members recognize that other members' success can be helpful and they develop optimism for their own improvement
- *Universality*—group members recognize that other members share similar feelings, thoughts and problems
- *Imparting information*—group members experience education or advice provided by the therapist or other group members
- *Altruism*—group members gain a boost to self-concept through extending help to other group members
- *Corrective recapitulation of the primary family group*—group members have the opportunity to reenact critical family dynamics with other group members in a corrective manner

- *Development of socializing techniques*—the group experience provides members with an environment that fosters adaptive and effective communication
- *Imitative behavior*—group members expand personal knowledge and skills through the observation of other members' self-exploration and personal development
- *Interpersonal learning*—group members gain insight about their interpersonal impact through feedback provided from other members
- *Group cohesiveness*—group members experience increased feelings of trust, belonging and togetherness
- *Catharsis*—group members experience a release of strong feelings regarding present and/or past experiences
- *Existential factors*—group members begin to accept responsibility for life decisions.

Both the Corey (2012) and Yalom and Leszcz (2005) stages or phases can apply to group play therapy. These need to be considered in light of developmental issues as well as theoretical perspective.

Stages in group play therapy may also be theoretically based. Examples of this may include stages in Adlerian play therapy (Kottman, 2011), Ecosystemic play therapy (O'Connor, 2000), and Experiential play therapy (Norton & Norton, 2002). Many theoretical approaches discuss stages or phases, and are adapted to group therapy—and can be accordingly applied to group play therapy, if so adapted. We would suggest that theoretical consistency is imperative, as discussed in the Preface and Chapter 1.

Assessing Progress in Group Play Therapy

Assessing progress and the related issue of readiness for termination is an important issue in any play therapy process. It is not always a process marked by precision, as both subjective and objective measures must be considered. It is nevertheless an important issue to consider.

Recognizing that there are developmental considerations, Haworth (1994) suggested the following guide in consideration of measuring progress in play therapy:

1. Is there less dependence on the therapist?
2. Is there less concern about other children using the room or seeing the therapist?
3. Can the child now see and accept both good and bad in the same person?
4. Have there been changes in attitude toward time, in terms of awareness, interest, or acceptance?
5. Has there been a change in his reactions to cleaning up the room—less concerned if he formerly had been meticulous or interest in cleaning up as contrasted to earlier messiness?
6. Does the child now accept self?
7. Are there evidences of insight and self-evaluation; does the child compare her former actions or feelings with those of the present?
8. Is there a change in the quality or amount of verbalization?

9. Is there less aggression toward, or with, toys?
10. Does the child accept limits more readily?
11. Have his forms of art expression changed?
12. Is there less need to engage in infantile (e.g., bottle) or regressive (e.g., water) play?
13. Is there less fantasy and symbolic play and more creative constructive play?
14. Has there been a diminution in the number and intensity of fears?

(p. 416)

Sweeney (1997) offers similar criteria in assessing progress, but makes the crucial point that questions such as Haworth's need to be considered both in the therapy setting and also outside of the playroom: "We should expect to see increased levels of independence in therapy and at home and school. We should also anticipate changes that are more global and generalized in the life of the child" (p. 146). Sweeney suggests the following measures:

• Increased ability to problem-solve
• Increased verbalization [although this should not be an agenda for the therapist]
• Greater willingness to experiment and explore
• Increase in self-worth and self-confidence, and corresponding decrease in shame and self-deprecation
• Decreased anxiety and depression
• Increased ability to organize and order things, and corresponding decrease in chaotic thinking and behavior
• Increased ability to express emotions and tolerate the expression of emotions by others
• Decreased aggression
• Decreased fear of confrontation, and corresponding increased willingness to negotiate
• Increased willingness to give and receive nurture
• Increased frustration tolerance
• Increased willingness to seek assistance
• Increased ability to make decisions
• Changes in creative expression, including stories, artwork, etc.

Landreth (2012) suggests similar indicators for assessing readiness for termination, which although comparable, offer further considerations. These apply to both individual and group play therapy, and although directed towards children, span all developmental levels. He frames these in the context of "self-initiated change within children" (p. 358):

1. Child is less dependent.
2. Child is less confused.
3. Child expresses needs openly.
4. Child is able to focus on self.
5. Child accepts responsibility for his own actions and feelings.

6. Child limits her own behavior appropriately.
7. Child is more inner-directed.
8. Child is more flexible.
9. Child is more tolerant of happenings.
10. Child initiates activities with assurance.
11. Child is cooperative but not conforming.
12. Child expresses anger appropriately.
13. Child has moved from negative-sad affect to happy-pleased.
14. Child is more accepting of himself.
15. Child is able to play out story sequences; her play has direction.

(pp. 358–359)

In terms of group play therapy, progress should be assessed in relation to the above noted indicators, as well as in regard to the presenting problem, intrapersonal and interpersonal functioning in the group process, and consistent with the group rationale noted in Chapter 1. When improvement is seen in group members related to the rationale for placement in a therapeutic play group, this should be considered in regard to progress and readiness for termination.

Conclusion

This chapter has explored general group play therapy procedures that are cross-theoretical and consistent with group play therapy interventions discussed throughout this book. Before moving on to the next chapter, which discusses structure and limit-setting in group play therapy, it has been imperative to consider the common operational elements reviewed in this chapter.

6   Structural and Relational Limit-Setting

Without limits there could be no therapy.

(Moustakas, 1959, p. 10)

Group play therapy is built on relationships, including relationships between children and relationships between children and therapist. Limits are inherent in all relationships. The ability to express personal boundaries while accepting the boundaries of others is critical to healthy relationships. The negotiation of these boundaries is limit-setting but the mutual agreement in respecting these boundaries is the relationship. Group play therapy should aspire to be an intervention that promotes, encourages, and structures for the growth of healthy relationships.

As in individual play therapy, a therapist attitude of permissiveness in group play therapy allows children an environment where all feelings and symbolic actions are accepted, allowing children the freedom to express all of their thoughts, feelings, and actions. Once fully expressed and accepted, children can then start to create new paradigms of thinking, relating, and acting. However, permissiveness does not extend to inappropriate or harmful behaviors, especially toward others. In group, play therapists set limits that will help children feel safe and learn to develop behaviors that will allow expression of self in appropriate ways. A group play therapist is adept at understanding when limits need to be set and how to effectively set them.

There are different historical views regarding how limit-setting is seen in the playroom. Moustakas (1959) believed that the setting of limits "becomes a warm, practical, living experience which enables the child to live freely and fully and enables a relationship between two persons to deepen and grow" (p. 11). Ginott (1961) recognized a less positive view of conflict in group play therapy, warning "Play therapy, particularly group play therapy, provides many opportunities for testing the stability of the therapist and for bringing even the most accepting adult to the brink of his endurance" (p. 128). Whether seen as an opportunity or challenge, limit-setting in group play therapy is almost always required, necessitating skillful execution by the therapist.

Purpose and Rationale for Limit-Setting

Moustakas (1959) conceptualized the meaning of limit-setting in the context of relationships with children. As the play therapist grows to understand that limits are integral and alive within each relationship, there is less need to emphasize rules to fit all children and all relationships. It is the limits within a relationship that define that relationship as unique. Because each child is unique and each therapist is unique, each relationship is unique. Because each relationship is unique, specific limits within that relationship will be unique. The temptation to hold the same rules for all relationships constricts the growth of that relationship and persons within the relationship. This conceptualization to limit-setting is abstract and may confuse a therapist regarding concrete problematic actions taking place in group play therapy. However, embracing the idea that the therapist has no real solutions for every problem that takes place in group play therapy and focusing on the relationship base of intervention helps therapists be more self-accepting and creative when challenges arise.

Although Ginott (1961) stressed the value of allowing children to symbolically or verbally express any feelings or thoughts, he cautioned against allowing all behaviors. He proposed six statements of rationale for setting limits in play therapy. They are summarized below.

> Limits direct catharsis into symbolic channels. Because children may wish to act out their feelings or thoughts in unacceptable ways, limits set by the therapist and accepted by the child encourage the child to find a symbolic way to express self. Symbolism will allow gratification of the child's need without violating societal rules.

> Limits enable the therapist to maintain an attitude of acceptance, empathy, and regard for the child. Child behavior that is hurtful or harmful to the therapist interferes with the therapist's ability to provide therapeutic conditions. By setting limits, the therapist can also feel safe in the relationship and provide acceptance to the child.

> Limits assure the physical safety of the children and therapist. The therapist is responsible for the physical safety of all people in the playroom.

> Limits strengthen ego controls. Through the verbalization of limits, children who have poor self-regulation or impulse control will internalize the externalized values presented by the therapist.

> Some limits are set according to societal rules or laws. Children cannot engage in some behaviors, such as sexual acting out with one another or the therapist, because it is against the law, in addition to being morally unacceptable.

> Some limits are set because of budget limitations. Therapists set limits on materials that are expensive or cannot be replaced quickly.

> (pp. 103–105)

Landreth (2012) elaborated on Ginott's list by adding a few more thoughts about the rationale for limit-setting. Limits are set to provide structure to play therapy so that children feel a sense of safety and security. An environment with no limits is likely to cause anxiety and insecurity, interfering with the therapeutic process. Limits anchor a play session to reality by providing a child with decision-making opportunities. By setting a limit such as pouring paint on the floor, the child is confronted with the reality of the situation and the further reality that this type of decision-making is regularly offered to the child outside of the playroom. Furthermore, by offering the reality that the child is faced with decisions each day, the practice of responding to limits facilitates the child's effective and enhancing decision-making, as well as practice with taking responsibility for actions.

Structuring for Successful Limit-Setting

Group play therapy is based on the assumption that children will modify behavior in exchange for acceptance (Ginott, 1982), thereby establishing a base understanding that children selected to participate in group have demonstrated some control over impulses or acting on others when emotionally distraught. The need for social acceptance inhibits verbal and physical aggression directed toward others. Hence, the selection process of choosing children to participate in group is the first step in structuring that affects future limit-setting. Children who are highly aggressive toward others, impulsive, or excessively defiant or oppositional are not candidates for group play therapy. When children who exhibit these behaviors are not selected for group intervention, this will be one step toward preventing frequent limit-setting.

Structuring the presentation of the playroom or group is another way to address future limits and establish clarity with the group. In more nondirective approaches, such as psychoanalytic or child-centered play therapy, the therapist will present the playroom in a way that emphasizes permissiveness while minimally addressing limits, such as: "In here, you may say anything you want, and you may do almost anything you want. If there is something you may not do, I will let you know" (Cochran, Nordling, & Cochran, 2010, p. 136) or "this is our playroom. And this is a place where you can play with the toys in a lot of the ways you would like to" (Landreth, 2012, p. 184). Landreth explained that by using the words "a lot," the therapist communicates that limits do exist but emphasizes permissiveness.

In other approaches, group play therapists may begin the limit-setting process with establishing group rules. The therapist may initiate the session with: "We will meet in this room for 30 minutes each week. The rules for the group are: (1) We do not hit, push, or throw; (2) We listen to each other when one person is talking…" and so on. When the therapist establishes rules at the initiation of the group, there is clarity that the therapist is in charge of the structure and will likely respond in the playroom in a way that maintains that structure. Another method of introducing limit-setting in group is to have the group members establish the rules. For this approach, the therapist opens group with: "The first thing we need to do is to establish rules that we all agree on. What are your ideas for group rules?" The therapist facilitates this process until group members come to consensus on what rules will be implemented in group. Again, the result of this process will be clarity between therapist and group members that there are limits that will need to be followed. However, this second process is more likely than the therapist-centered approach to engage members to take ownership of limit-setting when other group members break the rules.

When to Set Limits

Despite the effective or ineffective use of directive or nondirective structuring, limits will need to be set at some time in group play therapy. Ray (2011) introduced four questions that can help a therapist decide on when to set limits. In the following section, we will apply these questions to the case of group play therapy.

Is a child's behavior physically hurting self, therapist, or others? As listed in most literature on limit-setting in play therapy, physical harm is never acceptable in the playroom. The play therapist should not allow a child to hit, kick, scratch, choke, or behave in any such manner. Limits are set in these cases. However, group play therapy provides an opportunity for reflection on this particular question. When a child punches another child in group, the clear action by the therapist should be limit-setting. But what of situations that present differently? In group play therapy, it is common for children to physically struggle over the same toy or for one child to physically shove another child to get to a place or toy faster. In these cases, the call for limit-setting may not be as clear. A therapist might feel that it is beneficial to watch a child who has previously deferred to another child to show progress by continuing to keep his hands on the same toy that another child is grabbing. The therapist may choose not to intervene so that the child may experience this new way of asserting himself and figure out if it is a self-enhancing coping skill. When one child shoves another resulting in the child falling down, a therapist may choose not to intervene with limit-setting so that the shoving child can see the consequences of her actions, how she has hurt another by poor impulse control. Although these situations can be complicated, the therapist may want to rely on the relationship base for decision-making. By setting or not setting limits on specific behavior, will the children feel safe? Will they be allowed to continue to test out new ways of interacting? Will they feel empowered to keep making contact with each other and the therapist?

Will the behavior interfere with the provision of play therapy? The facilitation of group play therapy requires that children enter the room, stay in the room, and leave the room at the end of the session. Behavior that interferes with these structural elements of play therapy typically creates a need for limit-setting. This is especially challenging in group play therapy where one child may be unwilling to respond to the structure but other children are eager to comply. Group play therapy involves the movement of group members together. When children go to the playroom, they go as a group. When one goes to the bathroom, it is often necessary for the whole group to go. When they leave the playroom, they leave as a group. Play therapists are not wise to leave individual young children alone in the playroom or wandering the halls of a clinic or school alone. In most cases, the group effect works in favor of structuring. If one child does not want to go to the playroom, the other children who are waiting will encourage or pressure the child to go. If the therapist has selected members according to a demonstrated need for acceptance in exchange for behavior, peer pressure becomes an effective tool for limit-setting regarding structuring. Yet, in other cases, a therapist may struggle with structuring when one child needs to leave the room but others desire to stay, such as in bathroom breaks. In these situations, the therapist may cajole the other children to leave the playroom by promising a short break or extended minutes to make up for the break. Problems with leaving the playroom may require the assistance of a child's parent who removes the child from the playroom while the therapist says goodbye to the other children.

Will the behavior harm the continued use of the playroom for other clients? The intended and unintended destruction of materials and the playroom in the midst of group play therapy is common. The level of activity involved in nondirective approaches to play therapy invites mishaps and accidents. Group play therapists ensure that the playroom and materials are as indestructible and easily replaced as possible. When children are unaware of destruction caused by their behavior, a therapist may set a limit to raise awareness. For example, two children may start throwing paint on easel paper but as they become more excited, they start to splatter paint on the walls and floor. The therapist responds: "You guys are having a lot of fun, but the paint isn't for going on the wall or floor, you can keep putting it on the paper." However, when children become destructive in an intentional way, the therapist will want to point out the intention. An example would be two children who throw the toys on the floor and then start stomping on them. The therapist responds: "You guys are trying to break the toys but the toys aren't for breaking, you can stomp the Bobo." This limit addresses the intention of the child, not just the feeling, allowing the therapist to convey her acceptance of the children's desire to be destructive but limiting the behavior.

How will the child's behavior affect the relationship between therapist and child? In the case of group play therapy, a therapist would question the effect of the behavior of one child affecting the relationship between herself and others or between herself and the therapist. The answer to this question is related to the promotion of therapist acceptance of child, as well as the acceptance by other group members. This is also a difficult question in the application of group play therapy. Many behaviors beyond social norms will be acceptable to the therapist but not to other children. This is certainly one of the main purposes of using a group intervention. One goal of group is to help children develop coping skills when faced with rejection or disapproval of others. Some behaviors such as loudly passing gas or crying are accepted by the therapist in individual play therapy, but fellow child group members are likely to provide feedback of intolerability. This leads to the question of limits. The therapist may initiate a limit on behaviors that may interfere with therapist acceptance, but does the therapist initiate limits on behaviors that interfere with the group's acceptance? Tougher examples of these situations are in cases where a child continues to make a high pitch sound that irritates other group members, or deliberately moves closer to other group members to pass gas. In group play therapy, the hope is that the group provides feedback and the member begins to change. Cases where the child continues to alienate others even after receiving feedback require the therapist to question the need for a limit.

Another consideration for this point is verbal interaction between children. In individual play therapy, it is accepted practice that a therapist allows all verbalizations of a child. However, in group play therapy, this practice is questionable. Verbalizations such as cursing, name-calling, or using racial slurs are often limited in group play therapy because of their effects on children. These types of verbalizations may prevent a feeling of safety between children. In addition, some children who have not been exposed to certain types of language may learn words that are objectionable to their parents from other children in the group. We encourage group play therapists to heavily consider the consequences of allowing all verbal expression in the group environment.

The purpose of the four questions is to emphasize the subjectivity related to setting limits in group play therapy. There is not one set of limits that fits all groups. Through conceptualizing limits within the context of relationship, understanding the rationale for setting limits and asking questions of self-reflection, play therapists will be careful and effective in their ability to apply limit-setting in groups.

Although limit-setting is a subjective process, Ray (2011) suggested that there are a few limits that appear to be universal in the facilitation of play therapy. She worded them as definitive limits: (1) I, or others, are not for hurting; (2) You are not for hurting; (3) I, or others, are not for touching in private places; (4) In the playroom, you are not for touching in private places; (5) The walls are not for painting, gluing, throwing water on; (6) Sand is not for throwing; (7) Video equipment/two-way mirror is not for playing with; (8) Your clothes are not for taking off; (9) My clothes, or others', are not for taking off; (10) The playroom is not for peeing/pooping in; (11) My hair/clothes, or others', are not for cutting; (12) Your hair/clothes are not for cutting; and (13) Glue/paint is not for drinking.

Setting the Limit

There are several approaches to limit-setting with distinctive differences emerging from a nondirective or directive approach to group play therapy. In nondirective approaches, emphasis is placed on recognizing and accepting the child's feelings and intentions while placing restrictions on actions. The assumed outcome is that, in an accepting environment, children will utilize inner resources to create new, more self-enhancing, ways of handling conflict. In directive approaches, emphasis is placed on guiding children to build cognitive and behavioral skills to work through conflict.

NonDirective Approaches to Limit-Setting

Acknowledge, Communicate, Target.   Working from a child-centered approach to play therapy, Landreth (2012) developed the ACT model to limit-setting. The ACT model is built upon Ginott's (1961) initial recommendations for limit-setting, which included the reflection of the child's feelings, clear limits on specific acts, provision of alternatives, and helping the child facilitate his resentment of the limit. In Landreth's ACT model, A is to acknowledge the child's feelings or desires, thereby allowing a child an outlet for expression and sending the message the therapist understands and accepts the child's motivation. C is to communicate the limit in a clearly definitive statement. And T is target an alternative, which is to quickly redirect the child so that the child can still express the feeling but in an appropriate way. ACT is used the same in both individual and group play therapy, with the only difference being that sometimes the limit is directed toward multiple members of the group instead of just one. Examples include: "Tony and Ben, you are happy about throwing the toys against the wall (A) but toys aren't for throwing at the wall (C), you can throw the ball against the wall (T)." "Brandy and Christy, you are really mad at Madison (A) but Madison is not for throwing paint at (C), you can tell Madison you're angry (T)."

   In each of these examples, ACT is employed to share the therapist's understaning of the children's feelings or intentions, set a clear definitive limit, and provide an alternative to behavior that still meets the children's intentions. Through acknowledgement of feeling, children learn that there are words to express their desires and develop self-awareness of what feelings are tied to behaviors. Through communicating the limit, children learn they are in a safe environment where behaviors that are damaging are unacceptable and will be confronted. And through targeting alternatives, the therapist helps children begin to think of new behaviors that are appropriate but still allow expression (Ray, 2011).

   Choice-giving.   In most cases, ACT is effective and children will choose to willingly follow the limit and possibly enact the alternative. However, there will be times when ACT is not effective and the therapist needs to move to the next step of limit-setting, which involves choice-giving. A therapist decides to progress limit-setting to choice-giving when children have been offered an appropriate amount of time to rein-in impulses using ACT and they make a conscious choice to not follow the limit. When used in limit-setting, choice-giving adds the element of consequences to the child's awareness. To enact choice-giving, the therapist follows approximately three rounds of ACT with a choice that involves the giving up of a toy or material. Examples include: "Jen and Kim, if you choose to hit each other with the pots, you choose not to play with the pots." "Alex and Jorge, if you choose to throw paint on each other, you choose not to play with the paint."
   Limit-setting can be a tedious process with some children. When the goal is to help children learn to make their own enhancing decisions and not to just stop behavior, patience and persistence are the key elements. In every response, the therapist acknowledges the child's feelings, intentions, and ability to make the decision, yet clearly communicates the limit and the consequence of the limit. Once a therapist moves to choice-giving and a child chooses a consequence, it is the therapist's role to effectively follow-through on the consequence. It is possible that these interactions could take up to 15 to 30 minutes of a play session. I have experienced children who reenact the same scenario with different behaviors for an entire session. For example, shooting the therapist might be the first behavior to move to the choice-giving consequence, and then the child might move to throwing a ball at the therapist and the whole process starts over. These cases can be quite frustrating and I have heard therapists question the value of play therapy if these interactions pervade the session time. If children choose to use their play time engaging in multiple limit-setting interactions, then it becomes obvious that they are choosing to work through what is most problematic for them, making play therapy the environment where the child revisits the need for expression of self and limitation of such expression within a safe relationship.

Directive Approaches to Limit-Setting

Therapist-guided negotiation.   Kottman (2003) presented an Adlerian approach to limit-setting that differs from nondirective approaches yet still emphasizes the need for regarding the child as capable and creative. In her approach, there are four steps to limit-setting starting with the first step of stating the limit. Stating the limit requires the emphasis on rules of the playroom, such as "The rule is …" or "It's against the playroom rules to …" In the second step, the therapist recognizes the child's feeling or purpose of the behavior, similar to the acknowledgement step of Landreth's model. The therapist would say: "You're angry with me about …" or using metacommunication to verbalize the child's intention, the therapist might say: "You wanted to see how I would react when you threw that paint." For the third step, the therapist helps the child generate alternatives to the unacceptable behavior, often through negotiation. The therapist begins this step by presenting a statement such as "I bet you can think of another way to …" When the child responds, the therapist engages in negotiation or creating new more acceptable ideas. For example, when children suggest that they can pour ten buckets of water in the sand instead of an unlimited number, the therapist might respond by negotiating that ten is still too many. The therapist and children come to a consensus on what behavior would be acceptable. In the fourth step, the therapist and child enact logical consequences for breaking the agreed-upon limit. During the logical consequence step, the therapist engages children in the process of determining a reasonable consequence if the limit is broken. This step is also characterized by negotiation between therapist and child. Children may decide that if they pour too much water in the sand, they will restrict themselves from using the sand next session. As part of negotiation, the therapist would need to accept this consequence as reasonable and effective in preventing future problems with having too much water in the sand.

Problem-solving limit-setting.   Group play therapy offers the opportunity to involve multiple children in limit-setting and conflict resolution. As problematic behavior occurs in the playroom, the therapist can intervene to facilitate problem-solving. In four steps, problem-solving integrates cognitive processes of thinking through conflicts within the microcosm of the playroom where children can use new skills or attitudes toward interpersonal problems. As problems arise in the playroom, the therapist will bring attention to the problem in order to raise the children's awareness. The therapist may initiate the first step by saying: "When the two of you scream in the playroom, it disturbs other children in the clinic. I'd like for you to find another way to express yourself that won't interrupt others. What are all the ideas you can think of?" The next step is brainstorming in which the therapist encourages the children to think of as many alternatives as possible. The therapist can encourage this process: "That's an idea, what's another?" During the brainstorming phase, neither the therapist nor the children are allowed to censor any ideas. In this phase, all ideas are valid. Brainstorming is often enhanced by writing down all of the ideas on a chalkboard, white board, or large easel paper. Although the therapist should encourage ideas from the children, there might be a need for the therapist to suggest new ideas as the children become stuck in the process, especially if children are new to the problem-solving process. Once all ideas are written, the therapist initiates the third step, in which the therapist reviews each idea with the children to come to consensus on which idea seems like the best one. The therapist avoids guiding the consensus process to the therapist's desired outcome. Even if an idea does not seem that it will be successful, the therapist allows the children to decide. The therapist only places restrictions on ideas that cannot happen, such as children choosing to knock on each door of the clinic to apologize to clients. In the final step, the children commit to following the idea upon which they have agreed. In the future, if the consensus idea does not work, the therapist starts the process over from the beginning.

Case Example

Allison and Melissa are both 8 years old and in third grade at different schools. Both girls have participated in individual play therapy for over a year. Both girls come from single-mother homes with significant trauma in their backgrounds. Mothers independently report that both girls have no friends, are aggressive toward others at school, and seem generally unliked by others. In individual play therapy, the girls have been successful at working through their intrapersonal concerns and the relationships between mother and daughter are substantially improved. Yet, both mothers report social skill issues have not improved. The two therapists confer and decide that group play therapy seems to be the next step in the treatment process, agreeing that the two girls appear to be a good match.

In the initial stages of therapy, the girls are highly interactive and show an interest in playing with one another. They sometimes conflict over establishing who will lead the play, which results in raised voices but no physical aggression. In the sixth session, a conflict emerges, seemingly over a toy. Melissa has picked up a flute and begins to play.

ALLISON: Melissa, give me the flute. I want to play.

Melissa ignores Allison and keeps playing.

THERAPIST: Allison you really want to play with that, but Melissa you really want to play with it too.

ALLISON [stands by Melissa with arms crossed, becoming more agitated]: Give me it! Give me it!

THERAPIST: Allison, you're showing Melissa that you really want that flute.

Melissa begins to blow the flute loudly in Allison's face. Allison tries to grab the flute. Melissa quickly turns away.

THERAPIST: Melissa, looks like you're really trying to bug Allison.

ALLISON [to Melissa]: You're stupid. I hate you.

Allison goes to dart gun and begins shooting at wall. Melissa drops the flute and comes toward Allison.

MELISSA: Let me play.

ALLISON: No. You can't. [Allison then begins a sing-songy chant.] You can't play. You can't play. You're stupid and you can't play.

THERAPIST: Allison, you're trying to hurt Melissa as much as you can.

MELISSA [screaming]: You're evil. Evil. EVIL. [Melissa then heads toward Allison and shoves her to get the gun.]

Scenarios Using Different Approaches

ACT. In the ACT model, the therapist steps in between the girls to set the limit. Stepping in between the girls will stop the physical altercation and gain their attention to set the limit. The therapist says: "You are both angry, no one is for shoving in the playroom, you can tell each other that you are angry" or "You are both wanting to hurt each other, no one is for shoving in the playroom, you can shove the Bobo." In these responses, the therapist attempts to facilitate awareness and understanding of feelings and sets a very specific limit in response to the action. The therapist then attempts to provide an alternative on how to express emotion or let out physical energy. The therapist continues to use ACT with every physical altercation, assuring the physical safety of each girl. The purpose of using ACT in this case is to continually recognize and accept the girls' anger and attempt to hurt another person while sending responsibility back to the girls to create new ways of interacting without the therapist solving the problem for them. In this case, choice-giving would only be initiated in response to the use of toys to hurt each other. An example is: "If you choose to hit each other with the flute, you choose to not play with the flute."

Problem-solving. To initiate problem-solving, the play therapist intervenes by standing in between the girls.

THERAPIST: It is against the rules in the playroom to hit, shove, or hurt each other. I can see that you are really angry with one another. What are ways that you can express how mad you are without hurting each other?

MELISSA: She won't let me play.

ALLISON: She wouldn't let me play first. She's mean.

THERAPIST: You're both still mad at each other. What are some ways you can express how mad you are without hurting one another?

ALLISON: She could let me play when I ask.

MELISSA: She could ask nicely.

THERAPIST: So one way you could work it out is to ask nicely for what you want. What are other ways? [Therapist reaches to white board and writes down: "ask nicely."]

ALLISON: We could call a conference.

THERAPIST: What's a conference?

ALLISON: I could say I want a conference and then I would tell her what I want and she would tell me what she wants.

THERAPIST: Oh, that's an idea. What else?

MELISSA: You could tell us who gets the toy.

THERAPIST: So, I would be the one to decide for you. [Therapist has written all three ideas on the board. Because it is their first time engaging in problem-solving, the girls are out of ideas.]

THERAPIST: It looks like we have three ideas. Ask nicely, call a conference or have me decide. Which idea do you like the best?

MELISSA: I think we should call a conference when we get mad.

THERAPIST: So, Melissa, you like that idea. Allison, what about you?

ALLISON [proudly]: Duh, it was my idea.

THERAPIST: Let me make sure I understand. When either of you is angry, you're going to say "I call a conference" and then the other is going to say "okay". Then, both of you are going to say what you want to each other. Is that right?

ALLISON & MELISSA (nodding together): Yeah.

THERAPIST: So, we'll try out this conference idea the next time there is a problem. [Girls resume playing with no further incidents.]

In the problem-solving scenario, the therapist guides the girls through the process by reflecting, redirecting to the goal of problem-solving, and encouraging their ideas. The therapist trusts the girls to make the decisions regarding what they think will work best and then allows them the freedom to use the created method. If there is another future altercation and the girls choose not to use the conference idea, the therapist responds by saying "It looks like the conference idea is not working, what are some other ways you can figure out to get what you want without hurting others?" Through problem-solving, the girls can experience the process of thinking through their actions and considering consequences, an issue that both girls were struggling with in making friendships outside of the playroom.

Further Considerations in Group Limit-Setting

Therapist attitude.   In any limit-setting model, the therapist's attitude affects the outcome of the process. If the therapist believes that it is her job to control children's behavior, some children operating from a power and control orientation will respond with a need to oppose the therapist. This dynamic sets up a personal component to limit-setting which is rarely effective. As discussed in Kottman (2003), Landreth (2012), Ray (2011), and others, rules in the playroom should be approached from an objective stance. Limits are a regular part of being in the playroom and should be communicated casually to the child. Limits are not the therapist's choices or rules; they simply exist in the playroom and need to be shared with others who are new to the playroom (Ray, 2011). When approaching limit-setting, the therapist's tone of voice should be casual, but firm. A tone of voice initiated from a need for control will be perceived by some children as an invitation to struggle over who has power. Yet, a tone of voice that reveals fear of engagement in conflict will be perceived by some children as an invitation to manipulate or ignore. Therapists seek to maintain a strong sense of self, while letting go of a strong need to control others, in order to enact effective limit-setting.

Philosophy challenges (*Ray, 2011*).   The issue of limit-setting is directly related to the therapist's belief in the self-directed nature of children. There is no greater laboratory for experimenting with the question of a need for guidance for children versus a belief in their ability to positively self-direct their behavior than the group play therapy room. Nondirective play therapists embrace the belief that children have the ability to direct their behavior to positive outcomes, specifically in individual play therapy. However, in group play therapy, when a play therapist is forced to step in the middle of two children physically engaging in a fight, this belief system is challenged. The therapist must make the decision regarding the need for the introduction of a problem-solving method or the continued allowance of such aggression (while still stepping in when physical aggression is pursued) until the children tap into their positive nature and develop coping skills from an internal sense of doing what moves them toward self-actualization. Play therapists from directive approaches use limit-setting to explore children's ability to cognitively approach problem-solving and replace ineffective interpersonal skills with effective ones. Even coming from a directive approach, a play therapist struggles with the decision of how much to lead the process. Play therapists use the group play therapy experience as an opportunity to explore and clarify belief systems about children that help the therapist become a stronger, more effective agent for change.

Speed of group play therapy. Group play therapy is reserved for play therapists with extensive experience due to the need to respond rapidly to actions in the playroom. Rapid responses are typically needed in group play therapy limit-setting. Because children interact quickly and the therapist seeks to be fully present for each child as well as the group itself, limit-setting is challenging to say the least. Being present for one child may inhibit a therapist from seeing rising aggressive dynamics between other children. The therapist maintains a focused, yet alert, presence to all actions and dynamics taking place in the playroom. Experience with limit-setting in individual play therapy allows the group play therapist to feel more secure in the room and competent to respond to the quickly moving dynamics of group.

Support and self-care for the group play therapist. We do not suggest that play therapists should be fearful of engaging in limit-setting in play therapy. However, we highlight the extensive personal resources needed by a therapist to engage in group play therapy. Slavson (1999) warned: "The anxiety stimulated by the presence of other children and the support they give one another in their hostility toward the adult include hyperactivity and destructiveness seldom encountered in the play of one child" (p. 25). Both Slavson and Schiffer (1975) and Ginott (1961) emphasized the need for the therapist to be personally prepared, aware, and responsive to personal needs in order to be an effective group play therapist. The risk of countertransference is high in group play therapy due to the multiplicity of dynamics, such as a therapist overly aligning with a child who she perceives as victimized or initiating responses to fit in and be accepted by the group. Therapists benefit from staying continually aware of their personal processes and through consultation with other professionals. Additionally, therapists who engage in personal counseling can also explore implications of their personal histories on their practices with children.

7 Integrating Directive and Nondirective Group Interventions

There are more group play therapy interventions than can possibly be discussed in this book. There are many theoretical approaches (some of the main approaches were discussed in Chapter 2), and many more technical applications. We will take a brief look at some of these.

While some would argue that the play therapy world is divided into two primary camps—nondirective and directive—it is not this simple. Most play therapists take a somewhat integrative approach. In fact, we (the three authors of this book) have varied perspectives on play therapy and group play therapy. We would assert that this is part of the beauty of the play therapy landscape. Rather than taking a dogmatic position from any one perspective, we seek to provide a varied panorama, while also trying to be faithful to a robust clinical and ethical foundation.

In terms of play therapy theoretical orientation, Andrews (2009) found that "factors such as therapist personality, comfort level, clinical supervision and educational background influence therapist preference of play therapy treatment approach" (p. 42), and that "theoretical models are not as important as therapist personality when determining treatment approach" (p. 46). This is not necessarily negative, as long as theory choice is based on appropriate training and understanding.

We would argue that play therapists should be theoretically based, not theoretically bound. There are certainly clinicians who are *not* theoretically based, and those who *are* theoretically bound. As we reflect upon different approaches and interventions, we hope for the same balance and acceptance among therapists that we wish for our clients.

This chapter will consider both nondirective and directive approaches, look at integrating the two, and then follow this with a variety of group play therapy activities and techniques used by the authors.

Nondirective vs. Directive

The term nondirective is often used as a substitute or simultaneously with the term child-centered. Landreth (2012) gives a description of the nondirective approach to play therapy:

> Nondirective play therapy makes no effort to control or change the child and is based on the theory that the child's behavior is at all times caused by the drive

for complete self-realization. The objectives of nondirective play therapy are self-awareness and self-direction by the child. The therapist has a well-stocked playroom, and the child has the freedom to play as she chooses or to remain silent. The therapist actively reflects the child's thoughts and feelings, believing that when a child's feelings are expressed, identified, and accepted, the child can accept them and is then free to deal with these feelings.

(p. 34)

Building upon this, Landreth and Sweeney (1999) suggest: "Child-centered group play therapy is based on an abiding trust in the group's ability to develop its own potential through its movement in a positive and constructive direction" (p. 44). Landreth and Sweeney assert that the facilitator of a child-centered group does not actually apply techniques to promote group growth, suggesting that the leader and emerging therapeutic relationships in the group are the instruments for change.

Development in the child-centered approach is often talked about as a process of becoming, consistent with Rogers' (1951) premise. Child-centered group play therapy theory has been discussed in Chapter 2.

Kenney-Noziska, Schaefer, and Homeyer (2012) argue, however, that it is not really possible to be completely nondirective in play therapy, or completely directive. A nondirective therapist uses directive skills at times, and the directive therapist use nondirective skills. This point would be argued by most nondirective or child-centered play therapists.

There is, and perhaps will long be, some controversy between nondirective and directive approaches to play therapy. Shelby and Felix (2005), for example, briefly laud and then strongly repudiate nondirective play therapy as an effective intervention with traumatized children. Andrews (2009) suggests: "Some self-identified nondirective therapists expressed concerns that directive treatment approaches dismiss the importance of building a trusting relationship and may force children to confront issues they are not ready to face" (p. 44).

It is challenging to discuss "directive" approaches to play therapy and group play therapy, because this would encompass a wide variety of theoretical orientations and technical applications. Many of the theoretical approaches discussed in this book are considered directive, and many of the techniques discussed—including all of the techniques discussed below—are considered directive. It is probably best to consider nondirective and directive techniques on a continuum.

At the end of the continuum, on the nondirective side, would be Axline (1947) and Landreth (2012). On the other end of the continuum might be cognitive-behavioral play therapy (Knell, 2011), solution-focused play therapy (Nims, 2011), and posttraumatic play therapy (Shelby & Felix, 2005). It is almost impossible to assign specific places on any such continuum.

Kenney-Noziska et al. (2012) talk about black and white thinking in regard to the nondirective versus directive debate, arguing that it is inappropriate to "demonize" someone with an opposing orientation. They appropriately note that if this occurs, it precludes a rational discussion with people of differing theoretical approaches. There are numerous theoretical approaches on the directive–nondirective continuum. This leads to discuss an integrative approach.

Integrative

It is difficult to talk about an integrative approach in the field of play therapy, because it is equally challenging to do so in the field of psychotherapy. Although Prior's (1996) comments are almost two decades old and written in the context of object relations therapy, they ring true for today across all theories: "There is no agreed-upon model of conceptual understanding and therapeutic practice that most clinicians would adhere to, and that would form a framework for shared assumptions, practices, and interpretive ideas" (p. 5). He goes on to consider that many therapists struggle to integrate, "with little to guide them and certainly no comprehensive model with which to work" (p. 5).

There are increasing calls for further integration in the general field of psychotherapy, and more specifically play therapy. This is in part related to the disagreements about nondirective versus directive discussed above. Drewes (2011) asserts the following:

> In the field of play therapy, there is limited coursework, articles, books and workshops available to help play therapists in becoming more flexible and integrative. There are still some purists who feel being well grounded in one treatment approach and theoretical framework is satisfactory for the treatment of most clients. However, in recent years there has been a surge in interest, books, and training in blending play therapy with cognitive-behavioral therapy, which has helped move play therapists toward a more integrative direction.
>
> (p. 33)

Gil (2006) argues for an integrated approach when working with abused and traumatized children, noting that "Mental health professionals who pursue this approach must remain conversant with a variety of theories and approaches (both evidence-based and clinically sound), and have the ability to shift perspectives in order to maximize therapy opportunities for their clients" (p. 19). This applies to both individual and group play therapy, which Gil discusses in her 2006 text. She further argues that "Rigid therapy agendas or clinical biases, however, can limit or overwhelm child clients" (p. 15). This would be true for adolescent and adult clients as well.

Gil (2006) goes on to list general treatment principles she uses in the integrative treatment of abused and traumatized children. These are principles that apply to presenting problems for clients of all ages:

- Provide a child-friendly therapeutic setting in which children and their families receive timely and informed responses.
- Conduct a comprehensive assessment of each child and family, withholding assumptions and biases that might affect clinical goal setting and expectations for treatment outcome.
- Construct a genuine, respectful, trust-filled, earnest *relationship* with each child client and his or her family.
- Provide services within a coordinated multidisciplinary context that centers on the best interests of the child, while also maintaining an awareness of legal procedures, time frames, and outcomes.

- Ensure that all clinical procedures are sensitive to culture, gender, and developmental age and stage.
- Maintain a focus on contextual and systemic issues.
- Assist parents or other caretakers to understand and better manage their crisis situation and respond appropriately to their children.
- Provide therapeutic approaches and services that best match the learning styles of parents/caretakers and children.
- Make a balanced and realistic assessment of family strengths and vulnerabilities.
- Identify and engage someone in each child's life (in either the family or the larger community) who sees the child as important and who will maintain an active advocacy role for him or her.
- Offer an understanding of the limitations and difficulties of court-mandated treatment, and make attempts to restore a sense of control to parents/caretakers who may feel disempowered and overwhelmed by agency expectations.
- Finally, employ a team approach in which the limits of confidentiality are clearly understood by family members.

(pp. 60–61)

These principles allow for integration of both theory and techniques, within a context of clinical and ethical competency.

An integrative approach to group play therapy should be rooted in theory, which provides a platform for technical eclecticism. This creates an opportunity for employment of group play therapy across a broad range of presenting issues and/or diagnostic categories, as well as the developmental lifespan. Whether the words "integrative," "eclectic," or "prescriptive" are used—recognizing these are potentially polarizing terms—a theory grounded synthesis of approaches may be the way to move in individual and group play therapy.

Group Play Therapy Techniques

Several chapters in this book look at specific group therapy techniques, including expressive arts, sandtray, puppet play, and activity therapy. Other chapters consider specific populations, such as group play therapy in schools, for bereavement and loss, and for disaster response. The following will include a variety of group play therapy techniques that we have used across a variety of settings, and can be left to the clinical judgment of the group play therapist.

Kinetic Family/School Drawing

The Kinetic Family Drawing is an often used art therapy intervention that is used in a variety of ways (Burns & Kaufman, 1980), and can be used in a group setting. Essentially, clients are asked to draw a picture of their family, including themselves, doing something. A Kinetic School Drawing involves having clients drawing a picture of themselves at school, including a friend and a teacher, and doing something. It can be used with drawing materials (markers, paint, pencils), sandtray miniatures, clay, or other expressive items. Generally, this would be done in the context of parallel play, but can also be done as a group project.

Hollywood Director

This technique is just like it sounds. It requires three materials—a director's chair, a bullhorn, and a director/production slate (the rectangular board with scene numbers, and a hinged bar—used when the director calls out "Action"). It's always helpful to have real materials, but improvised materials work fine. For example, using masking tape on the back of one chair with the word "Director" marked on it, an empty paper towel tube (to serve as a bullhorn), and a piece of cardboard to serve as the director/production slate.

Each group member has the opportunity to direct the rest of the group members in a scripted scene, relevant to the therapeutic focus of the group. The therapist must be a proficient timekeeper, ensuring that every group member has the opportunity to take on the role of director. This may be challenging to do all in one group session, depending on time constraints. It can be done over a series of sessions.

This technique is simply a variation of drama therapy. The script can be provided by the therapist, or can be made up by the group or by individual group members. It can also be improvisational. If the group members make up the scripts, the therapist has the responsibility to ensure that no member of the group is in any way denigrated. The benefit of each person being the director is that each person has the role of being in control and thus empowered.

Scribble Technique

This technique is mentioned in Chapter 8, but is mentioned here in more detail. Most people know how to scribble, and this simple technique can be simple and nonthreatening. Kramer (1993) and Oaklander (1978) discuss this technique in greater detail. There are several variations to this activity.

Group members can each be given an identical piece of paper with an identical scribble on the paper. They are each asked to make a drawing out of the scribble. Upon completion, the drawings are shared with the group

Group members are asked to select a single color marker. On a large piece of paper (2′–3′ × 4′–6′), the therapist makes the "first" scribble, and the group members are asked to successively add to scribble until the picture is done. This will essentially be the point at which no one has anything further to add. It should be noted if any group member dominates this activity (which can be a subject of group discussion, at the therapist's judgment). The therapist should make the first scribble, unless this activity is repeated so that each group member has the opportunity to make the initial scribble.

An adaptation of the above technique involves group members taking a single sheet of paper, writing their name on the paper, and making an initial scribble. The papers then are handed around the group until each group member has had the opportunity to add the scribble of every group member. Each group member should work with a single color, so that each contribution can be identified. Titles of these projects can be decided upon by the originator or the group.

Oaklander (1978) suggests a scribble activity that can be adapted for use in groups that involves body movement. Each group member is asked to move (stand up, sit on the floor, etc.), close their eyes and imagine a scribble/picture as large as their hands can stretch. They are then asked to draw the scribble in the air. It may be helpful for them to hold a marker in hand to assist with this imaginary process. It may also be helpful to give a short time limit to this part of the exercise, to limit those members who could continue for a long time and to decrease the anxiety of those who might be less comfortable with the activity. Remind the group members that no one else can see their movements, as all eyes are closed. [Therapists should be aware—some people, especially trauma victims, may be uncomfortable with closing their eyes.] Group members are then asked to draw what they have imagined on a piece of paper. The drawings are then shared with the group.

Sculpting (with Play-Doh® or clay)

Sculpting can be a powerful sensory and kinesthetic intervention. The sensory and malleable nature of clay seems to have a power to touch deep psychological places. It is up to the therapist what type of material to use. Play-Doh® has advantages and disadvantages. Its color and texture can be inviting, but it is not as moldable as potter's clay. Potter's clay is easier to mold and more sensory/sensual than Play-Doh®, but is generally mono-color and can be quite messy.

Children, adolescents, and adults generally enjoy the process, but may be turned off by the potential messiness of working with clay. It is helpful to have wet rags or paper towels, premoistened towlettes (diaper wipes work well!). It is also helpful to remind group members that both clay and Play-Doh® tend to dry up and crumble. Clients are also encouraged to participate if the therapist demonstrates by using the material.

The materials needed include: Play-Doh® or potter's clay, plastic or paper plates (upon which to make the sculpture), water, paper towels/rags/premoistened towlettes, and simple sculpting tools [wire clay cutter, putty knives, cheese cutter, rubber mallet (and/or potato masher), garlic press, pencil/straw (for poking holes), etc.]. The manufacturers of Play-Doh® have multiple accompanying sculpting toys if this material is selected.

Adequate space for each group member is needed. If adequate table-top space is unavailable, a vinyl tablecloth for the floor works fine. It is also possible to use individual plastic trays (cafeteria style) for each group member. This can be particularly helpful for cleanup purposes as well.

Instructions can be as directive or nondirective as the therapist chooses. It is often helpful to have group members initially handle the material (squeezing, pounding, poking, etc.) prior to any specific instructions. This can be done with eyes opened or closed. Often, handling the material with closed eyes can be anxiety reducing.

Group members are then asked to make a sculpture, which can be specific (for example, asking group members to make an animal which represents how they feel about themselves), or general (make anything they desire). Members can also be asked to think about a particular issue—if the group is focused on a topic, this would be the obvious choice—and then make a sculpture that fits with their emotional response to the issue. The sculpted creations can be taken home by the group members, or saved by the therapist for future group activities. These creations can have powerful meaning for the clients.

Beach Ball Game

This technique was developed by Post Sprunk (2010) for use with families, but works quite well with groups. It involves using a small beach ball that has 4–6 colors. Group members stand or sit in a circle, and the beach ball is tossed to a different group member. The one who catches the ball notices which color his or her right thumb is touching on the ball at the time of the catch. Sprunk provides a series of questions to be used corresponding with each color.

- Red
  - My family likes to…
  - My family is proud of me when…
  - I feel bad if my family…
  - I let someone in my family make me feel…
  - I wish my family…
- Orange
  - My happiest memory with my family is…
  - I need…
  - I feel hurt when…
  - I would not like to have…
  - I'm expected to…
- Blue
  - I love to give…
  - Once someone helped me…
  - When something is hard for me I…
  - I don't like to…
  - I would hate to lose…
- White
  - I like the way…
  - Something I appreciate about my family is…
  - I'm sad when…
  - I get angry when…
  - My mother and I like to…
- Green
  - I just love to…
  - I'm the kind of person…
  - My father thinks I…
  - If someone loves you, they…
  - At home I really like…

The questions can be changed, depending on the group and the therapeutic intent. This exercise works as an effective way to increase communication in group process.

This technique is one of dozens in Liana Lowenstein's (2010) book, *Creative Family Therapy Techniques*—many of which can be adopted for use with groups of all ages.

The "Would You Rather?®"Game

Would You Rather® is a game produced by the company Zobmondo. The game is based on asking game players opposing questions—both silly questions, and both not necessarily positive choices to make. Some sample questions from the *Would You Rather®* game include:

- Would you rather…
  - Have eyeballs the size of golf balls—OR—teeth the size of computer keys?
  - Be stuck in a tiny room at night with your dad while he is sound asleep and snoring like a loud motorcycle—OR—be stuck inside that same room alone all day with a huge pile of your dad's dirtiest socks?
  - Know your own future—OR—know the future of your friends and not be able to tell them?
  - Shave your head and eyebrows bald for a year—OR—wear a really good looking clown wig for a year?
  - Always have a thick white coating of spit on your tongue—OR—always have really sweaty palms?

In the process of group play therapy, the therapist can use preselected and appropriate questions from the game, or can make up questions, either generally relating to the group or pertinent to a particular client. It would be important not to ask for too much self-disclosure. Some sample made-up "therapeutic" questions include:

- Would you rather…
  - Have your parents shout at you all the time—OR—give you the silent treatment?
  - Wear your sister's clothes to school—OR—clean her bathroom with only a toothbrush and your spit?
  - Read mom's (dad's) mind when she/he is mad at you—OR—be forced to listen to their favorite music for one week?
  - Sell your own toys and give the money to your brother—OR—be stuck talking to no one else but him for a year?
  - Be caught by your kids dancing naked with your partner—OR—have to agree with your spouse on *every* financial expenditure?

The game provides a scoring system, but this is not necessary in the group process.

Fortune Cookie Sentence Completions

Sentence completion exercises are common therapeutic interventions—either in session or as homework. This is simply a variation, using fortune cookies. If working with children, it is best to check with parents beforehand, regarding any objections or possible food allergies. The printed fortunes in fortune cookies are simply removed, and replaced with sentence completion phrases.

It may be best to begin with some less threatening sentence completions, such as:

- My favorite color is…
- My favorite food is…
- If I could be an animal, I'd be…
- My favorite television show is…
- If I could change the color of my hair…

Then, the sentence completions could become a little more probing, such as:

- The thing that really makes me mad is…
- People say I am…
- I feel bad when…
- I get in trouble because…
- I can't…
- I get scared and worried when…

Group Art Activity

Similar to Landgarten's (1987) group/family art exercise, this intervention can be used as an initial screening device, to facilitate group interaction, or to assess individual and/or group dynamics. The materials needed include large (2′–3′ × 4′–6′) sections of paper and a set of colored markers, preferably with no duplication of colors. Two general types of interventions can be used.

Group members are instructed that they will be working together on two drawings. This may involve two drawings during the same session, or one drawing each for two successive sessions. The paper can be taped to the wall or placed on a tabletop. This facilitates easy access to the paper by all group members.

For the first drawing, the group members are asked to select a color and draw a picture together on the paper. These instructions should include that members may not trade colors and may not talk or signal each other during the completion of the art activity. They are free to finish at different paces, and should signal their being finished by capping the markers. The therapist remains in an observer role.

Following group completion, members may again talk, and are asked to title the picture. This title process should be a collaborative effort.

The second picture includes the same instruction, but this time the group members are free to talk during the art exercise. Group members are again asked to not trade colors.

The following questions [adapted from Landgarten (1987)] are helpful considerations:

- Who initiated the picture and what was the process that led up to this person making the first mark on the page?
- In what order did the rest of the members participate?

- Which members' suggestions were utilized and which were ignored?
- What was the level of involvement on the part of each person?
- Which participants remained in their own space versus those who crossed over?
- Did anyone "wipe out" another member by superimposing his or her image on top of someone else?
- What roles did each group member assume?
- Did the members take turns, work in teams, or work simultaneously?
- Where are the geographical locations of each person's contribution?
- How much space did each person occupy?
- What was the symbolic content of each person's contribution?
- Who acted as initiators—who followed or reacted?
- Were emotional responses made during the activity?

Each group member can be identified in the picture(s) by the color selected. The completed products provide a picture of individual and group dynamics. The therapist can use this material to comment on these dynamics without interpreting. It is helpful to remember that the interpretation of the group and the group members is far more important than the interpretation of the therapist. Additionally, it is helpful to comment (reflect) rather than question, as questions call for cognitive responses, often in the midst of distinct affective material.

Picture/Photo Collage

Collage work can be engaging and nonthreatening for group members as pictures and photos can easily be selected for their personal meaning, and there is obviously less need for artistic ability than with other art interventions. Magazine pictures are easy to collect and share with clients (an adequate supply of magazines from a variety of venues is important), and can express a wide variety of feeling states. Photos—either brought in by clients or taken in session by the therapist and/or group members—can also be powerful anchors or additions to the collage process.

If photos are used, the process should be structured and monitored. If photos are brought from home, the therapist should instruct about common photo size (e.g., 4″×6″), photo subject (the group members themselves, family members, favorite pet, etc.), and any restrictions or prohibitions. If photos are taken in session, it is advised to get written consent (particularly from parents). Photos taken during session should also have some degree of structure, balancing a consistent experience with group members' individuality. It may be helpful to take photos of group members with the instruction to have them pose however they wish in order to represent their self-concept, their current affective state, or how they feel about a specific issue. Creating a collage around such pictures can be a powerful therapeutic experience. An instant camera (e.g., Polaroid) or a digital camera with instant download and printing capability will be necessary.

Basic collage materials needed include: a variety of magazines, crayons, colored markers, paints, glue, scissors, tissue paper, ribbons, yarn, and basic poster board. Other materials may also be used, including colored tape, fabrics, construction paper, leaves, feathers, etc. The therapist should supply basic materials, although group members can bring in additional materials.

Whether or not a photo is used to anchor the collage, it is essentially a self-portrait for each group member. The group should work simultaneously on their collage projects, and are free to talk and share materials. Its creator should title the final product and group members are encouraged (not compelled) to share with the group how their "portrait" represents who they are.

Play/Sandtray Genograms

While genograms are most often done in family therapy, they are powerful when used in the group context as well. It is usually done in a parallel fashion, with group members constructing their own. It essentially involves the creation of a family tree, using sandtray miniatures to represent family members. Genograms are creative "maps" to family structure and dynamics. The group play therapist simply asks group members to select one or more miniatures that show their thoughts and feelings about every member of the family, including them. This should be done on a large piece of paper, rather than using the sandtray. The therapist can provide guidance for group members drawing the genogram outline—using the customary squares [for males] and circles [for females], as well as the lines that correspond to the family relationship. Miniatures are then selected to be placed on top of the squares and circles (Homeyer & Sweeney, 2011).

Usually, group members will choose miniatures simultaneously, as this can prevent the self-consciousness that can develop if members are compelled to select while others are watching. After the selection, the therapist facilitates discussion of the miniatures selected. Group members are invited to be a "tour guide," taking other group members on a tour of their own family. They are free to go into as much or little detail as they choose. The therapist should keep aware of time management issues, and allow equal time for all group members. A great deal of insight can be gained through the processing of chosen miniatures.

This genogram using sandtray miniatures can also be extended to another part of the genogram process. In traditional genograms, various line configurations and symbols are used to depict relationships (e.g., three parallel lines indicates enmeshment, a jagged line indicates conflict, etc.). With this adaptation, group members can also select miniatures to represent their perspective on the nature of their own family relationships (Homeyer & Sweeney, 2011). An example might be the selection of a miniature wall, which would be very telling about how one family member perceives relationship with another.

Conclusion

Following a discussion about nondirective, directive, and integrative work in play therapy, we have provided a small sampling of group play therapy techniques that we have used. There are many more, some of which are discussed in other chapters. Some suggested resources for many more play therapy techniques that can be adapted for groups may be found in: *Active Interventions for Kids and Teens* (Ashby, Kottman, &

DeGraaf, 2008); *Group Play Interventions for Children* (Reddy, 2012); *Assessment And Treatment Activities for Children, Adolescents, and Families* (Lowenstein, 2008); and *101 More Favorite Play Therapy Techniques* (Kaduson & Schaefer, 2004).

In consideration of integration of theory and practice, Kenney-Noziska et al. (2012) provide an important reminder for play therapists:

> Sound application of best practices would infer that when developing a treatment intervention for a particular client, play therapists must consider not only their preferred theoretical approach, but also empirical evidence regarding the most effective treatments for the presenting problem, as well as client variables, such as treatment preferences and personality.

(p. 246)

8   Expressive Arts in Group Play Therapy

Play therapists who imagine their new clients are three young children named Vincent Van Gogh, Frida Kahlo, and Salvador Dali will be motivated to learn about expressive arts in group play therapy. Perhaps Vincent's mother may have sought group play therapy because he isolated himself in a room for weeks at a time followed by bursts of energy in which he ran through fields of flowers. Frida's mother may have wanted group play therapy because she had a poor self-image and bouts of anger, particularly after she survived a serious traffic accident. Salvador's mother may have desired group play therapy because his peers perceived him as eccentric and bizarre in his behavior and drawings. All three mothers may have requested expressive arts therapy due to their children's unique interest in art. How do play therapists prepare for expressive arts in group play therapy sessions? What materials are needed? Should the session be nondirective or directive? What activities should be used? How should conflict between children be handled? This chapter will prepare play therapists to use expressive arts in group play therapy, whether their clients are future artists or typical children.

Definitions

Since there is considerable overlap between play therapy and art therapy with children (Rubin, 2010), it is helpful to begin with definition of terms. Play therapy and group play therapy are defined in Chapter 1. Yet, it is helpful for play therapists to explain the following terms to children, parents, teachers, and other stake holders.

Art is a traditional healing activity that has been utilized across cultures from the beginning of human existence (McNiff, 2009). Historical examples of art were identified by Rubin (2010):

> Prehistoric artists who drew animals on the walls of caves or who carved fertility figures, Egyptian painters of protective symbols on mummy cases, Tibetan Buddhist creators of sand mandalas, African carvers of ritual masks, Byzantine painters of sacred icons, Ethiopian artists who drew on parchment healing scrolls, Zuni carvers of magic fetishes—all represent historical antecedents of modern art therapy.
>
> (p. 50)

The healing capacity of art is reflected in Pablo Picasso's (n.d.) statement that "the purpose of art is to wash the daily dust of life off of our souls."

Artistic versus Creativity is a needed distinction to mitigate the performance anxiety that children may have when art materials are presented. Artistic implies having a special talent in depicting images through art material. Clearly, Vincent Van Gogh, Frida Kahlo, and Salvador Dali were such people. Yet, creativity is a universal characteristic that can be elicited within each person. Wadeson (2010) writes "creativity is not the same as art. Not everyone is capable of becoming a great artist. But all people are creative, no matter how limited" (p. 5). Explaining this difference creates a sense of unconditional positive regard leading to psychological freedom so children can fully express self, experiences, and perceptions in art.

Art therapy is a field in which trained art therapists help clients "use the particular creative medium of art expression to advance the larger creativity of making their own lives meaningful (Wadeson, 2010, p. 5). The American Art Therapy Association (2012) defines art therapy as follows:

> Art therapy is the therapeutic use of art making, within a professional relationship, by people who experience illness, trauma, or challenges in living, and by people who seek personal development. Through creating art and reflecting on the art products and processes, people can increase awareness of self and others; cope with symptoms, stress, and traumatic experiences; enhance cognitive abilities; and enjoy the life-affirming pleasures of making art.
>
> (p. 1)

Expressive Arts, in contrast to art therapy, is a therapeutic modality used by trained mental health professionals to facilitate the process of using art media for healing. The *process* of creating and reflecting is emphasized rather than the art *product*. Some view expressive arts therapy as encompassing modalities beyond art. "Expressive arts therapy is the practice of using imagery, storytelling, dance, music, drama, poetry, movement, dreamwork, and visual arts together, in an integrated way, to foster human growth, development, and healing" (Atkins, 2002, p. 3). Each of these expressive arts therapy modalities are characterized by self expression, active participation, imagination, and mind–body connection (Malchiodi, 2005).

Art supplies needed for expressive arts within group play therapy include the following:

- Surfaces (i.e., paper, canvases, cardboard, wood)
- Drawing materials (i.e., colored pencils, charcoal, markers, crayons)
- Painting materials (i.e., watercolors, tempera, oils, acrylics, finger paint)
- Modeling materials (i.e., clay, modeling doughs, Model Magic)
- Three-dimensional construction (i.e., papier-mâché, wood, rocks, yarn, pipe cleaners, fabric, plastic, foam, beads, feathers, etc.)
- Tools (i.e., scissors, brushes, knives, staplers, string, tape, glue) (Rubin, 2011).

Art materials range from things easily controlled like markers, magazine pictures, pipe cleaners to less controlled such as paint and wet clay. Play therapists need to select materials and activities based on their clients' developmental level and perceptual-motorskills. For example, finger paints may be more suited for younger children than oils.

Process in expressive arts is the activity of reflecting on the "*creation* of meaning, not discovery of meaning" (Wadeson, 2010, p. 3). It is not the product, but the process of accessing creativity imbedded deep within the psyche that promotes healing. The purpose of the process is to allow each child and then the group as a whole to achieve understanding through the integration of the personal and universal. The process helps each child to explore "me" and the group to explore "we."

Group play therapists create a safe place where subtle aspects of meaning can emerge throughout the process. Process is not magic, but rather "a flowering of germinating images and techniques" (Wadeson, 2010, p. 7). Rubin (2011) describes the process of art therapy as involving five components of (a) exploring the materials, (b) incubating and organizing, (c) reinforcing creative behavior, (d) being open-minded and flexible, and (e) observing the process. Throughout these components, the play therapist honors each group member's creative process. "What is essential is that you have sufficient respect for the person's creative process not to interfere with its organic evolution" (Rubin, 2011, p. 18).

Rationale

The rationale for using expressive arts in group play therapy is multi-faceted. First, art allows expression of imagery from dreams, fantasies, or experiences that are preverbal, traumatic, or deeply private (Wadeson, 2010). Images are often beyond logical verbal expression, particularly for children who are in concrete operations of cognitive development. Yalom (1989) elaborated on why images are communicated better through art rather than language.

> First there is the barrier between image and language. Mind thinks in images but, to communicate with another, must transform image into thought and then thought into language. That march, from image to thought to language, is treacherous. Casualties occur: the rich, fleecy texture of image, its extraordinary plasticity and flexibility, its private nostalgic hues—all are lost when image is crammed into language
>
> (p. 180).

For example, the image of the portrait of Dali is worth a thousand words in illuminating his personality (see Figure 8.1).

A second rationale for expressive arts is that it decreases children's defenses and hesitation for self exploration. Like adults, children may feel embarrassed to express thoughts, feelings, and fantasies. Expressive arts allow for unexpected things to burst forth, surprising even the creator (Wadeson, 2010). The art product of picture and sculpture gives voice to children's unconscious, whispering to be integrated into consciousness. For example, an 8-year-old boy drew his hero flying through the air shouting "to the rescue" to a woman at the bottom of his picture. Upon reflection the boy was surprised by how much the woman resembles his deceased mother. The art process

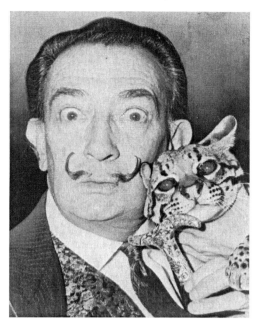

Figure 8.1 Salvador Dali with ocelot and cane. (Roger Higgins, 1965). Library of Congress. New York World-Telegram & Sun Collection (http://hdl.loc.gov/loc.pnp/cph.3c14985). No copyright restriction known.

revealed his longing to have been strong enough to rescue his mother from death. This insight softened his compulsion to prove his strength in the playroom by bossing around other children.

A third benefit of expressive arts is objectification via the production of a tangible product (Wadeson, 2010). Children may find it easier to relate to something concrete and tangible than to something as abstract as the "self." A projected image onto an object that children can touch and see is much easier for them to understand. For example, when a child holds her clay sculpture of a bird with a broken wing, she can readily explain the bird's sad feelings of not being able to fly with other birds. Eventually, the child may come to identify with the sculpture and recognize her own sadness related to chronic illness.

A fourth benefit is permanence of expression. Art products are permanent reminders of a moment in time and serve as a historical marker for subtle progress over time (Wadeson, 2010). Reviewing art products from months prior may reveal patterns such as fewer images of anger in comparison to the here and now. Noticing such changes over time is encouraging to children and play therapists. In addition, the permanence of an art product captures children's affect and thought in a way that is difficult for parents or teachers to deny. For example, when a child draws a picture of a witch to portray his teacher, the permanent object may prompt the teacher to engage in deeper self-reflection rather than attempting to filter or explain away the child's words.

Fifth, expressive arts allow for analysis of spatial relationship. Pictures can succinctly display "the closeness and distance, bonds and divisions, similarities and differences, feelings, particular attributes, context of family life, and so forth" (Wadeson, 2010, p. 13). It would be next to impossible for a young child to explain such characteristics about his or her family in words as clearly as in a picture. It is uncommon for children to even think about such characteristics. Yet expressive art reveals them in a manner that can bring forth deeper understanding of self in relation to others. For example, a picture in which step siblings are holding hands with father and mother in the center of the page while the client is depicted in the corner with the dog reveals the depth of isolation that the child feels.

Sixth, expressive art releases creative and physical energy. Fine motor and gross motor movement moves blood through the body that causes energy (Wadeson, 2010). Art activities utilize the creative, right hemisphere of the brain, causing blood to flow to a different part of the brain than is usually used in school classrooms. This release of creative and physical energy brings pleasure to children, thereby motivating them to continue in therapy.

A seventh rationale for expressive arts is enhancement of self-esteem. Children will discover new aspects of self as they express self through this safe, nonjudgmental process (Wadeson, 2010). This sense of mastery will increase self-esteem. They may even receive admiration and appreciation from other group members. The review of progress from beginning art projects to ending may bring relief and gratitude from parents and teachers.

A final rationale is that expressive arts with groups of children have been successful in treating numerous presenting problems, including anxiety related to hospitalization (Rollins, 2008), abuse and neglect (Gil, 2006; Malchiodi, 2008), Post Traumatic Stress Disorder (Carey, 2006; Hansen, 2006), grief and loss (Wakenshaw, 2002), Autism Spectrum Disorders (Gallo-Lopez & Rubin, 2012), and preadolescents with adjustment problems (Bratton & Ferebee, 1999). In fact, the use of expressive arts in group play therapy is a common strategy that has been widely implemented for decades (Kaduson & Schaefer, 1997).

Preparation for Expressive Arts

Preparing for expressive arts requires play therapists to consider group member selection, personal experience with art, physical space, goals, and roles.

Group Member Selection

Group member selection is critical to success. Play therapists must ensure group members are similar in age (i.e., within 2 years of each other), developmental level, presenting issues, and abilities to function in a group (Chapman & Appleton, 1999). Also, children need to be screened for allergies such as latex or physical limitations such as ability to work clay. The number of children in the group should match the play therapist's ability to successfully assist each child with art materials. The standard number of eight members per group may be reasonable for older elementary school children who follow directions readily. However, a more reasonable group size for younger children who are impulsive or limited in their cognitive ability would be three or four. The minimum number required for a group is two children.

Personal Experimentation

Play therapists are advised to engage in art activities and experience each material personally before asking children to do so. This personal experimentation of creating and processing the art material will increase play therapists' empathy of potential frustrations or surprises in art projects. Personally knowing the depth of insight expressive arts can bring gives play therapists confidence in the process. This experience also gives knowledge of time frames for engaging in and cleaning up the activity.

Physical Space

Enough physical space is needed so each child can safely explore and work with art media. At least 2´×2´ of working space is needed for each child as well as the play therapist. Art materials should be organized in bins and shelves to prevent children from being overwhelmed or over stimulated. Too much material and clutter can impede the creative process because excessive material can be distracting from the imagination. Tables and chairs should be arranged with easy access to art materials so the creative process is not hindered by excessive moving back and forth. Protective barriers to prevent stains on tables and floors can be created via paper or plastic covers that are taped down. Smocks or bibs in varying children's sizes should also be available to protect children's clothes.

Goals

Goals for each child and the group may vary depending on the nature of the group. Groups to resolve short-term specific issues such as a disaster recovery may have individual goals of emotional stabilization and not need goals of group cohesion. In contrast, groups for long-term therapy in settings such as a school or community clinic may have goals for each individual (i.e., anger management, social skills, bereavement) as well as group goals of cohesion and social support. These long-term groups need to develop trust and reliance through cooperative projects to achieve group cohesion.

Roles

The role of the play therapist in an expressive arts group may range from being a facilitator to being a strong leader, depending on the type and size of the group (Wadeson, 2010). In either case, the role entails being a role model of acceptance and respect for others. Another role is to be a witness to the expressive arts process. Finally, as a group play therapist, the role is to create a group climate where members learn to encourage and nourish each other rather than solely relying on the therapist.

Expressive Arts in Nondirective Group Play Therapy

Humanistic approaches to play therapy, particularly Psychoanalytic, Jungian, Person-Centered, Adlerian, and Gestalt tend to use a nondirective approach to expressive arts (Rubin, 2010). In these approaches, the group play therapist places carefully selected expressive art materials, appropriate for the group's age and developmental level, next to toys in the playroom. Children are free to explore the art materials and use them in most of the ways they choose in their own time. Some children may begin the session with an art activity of his or her choosing while others may do so in the middle of the session and still others not at all. This nondirective process is illustrated in the following CCPT dialogue of two 5-year-old girls from different families who both experienced a divorce.

PLAY THERAPIST: This is our playroom and you can play with all the toys and art materials in most of the ways you like.

ABBY: I'm playing with the mommy and baby [dolls] but not the daddy [said in anger].

CATHY: I'm going to paint!

PLAY THERAPIST: Abby, you've decided to play with just mommy and baby, but you're angry with daddy. Cathy, you are excited to paint.

ABBY: [Mommy doll gives baby doll a bottle].

CATHY: [Paints a tall smiling figure and a small figure with no mouth].

PLAY THERAPIST: Abby, the mommy is taking care of baby. Cathy, the tall one is smiling, but the shorter one is not.

CATHY: The short one can't talk or smile.

ABBY: Maybe she is mad at her daddy.

PLAY THERAPIST: Abby, you think she could be mad at daddy. Cathy, you can decide what the reason is.

CATHY: I guess she is mad at her daddy, but she can't talk about it.

PLAY THERAPIST: You both know what it is like to be mad at and hurt by daddy. Sometimes it seems you can't talk about it, but in here you can choose to talk or play about it if you want. You both have your own choice.

In the dialogue above, the child-centered play therapist communicated that each child was free to lead their play. She also tracked play behavior, reflected feelings, facilitated understanding, and linked their experiences for a sense of support and empowerment.

An option for nondirective groups is to use expressive arts to de-escalate group chaos or conflict. For example, Chapman and Appleton (1999) recount directing several preschool children to sit at the table to draw circles fast and then slow in an attempt to calm them down when they became too chaotic. I (Baggerly) have also used directed expressive arts activities with preadolescent boys who were intentionally excluding a member from the group. In this case, I asked the boys to sit down and draw their own picture of the group session. I prompted each member to tell about their picture and to state the thoughts and feelings of each figure in the picture. Each boy depicted the excluded boy as much smaller than the others and in the corner of the paper. When prompted, they identified the excluded boy as sad and lonely. Then I asked each boy to draw a picture of the group with members being kind to each other. Each boy shared figures of equal size closer to the middle of the paper. I affirmed their ability to create their own world and invited them to continue playing with the remaining time. The dominant boys made an effort to include the boy who previously was excluded.

Throughout the course of nondirective play therapy, children's spontaneous art can be used as a measure of progress. For example, two 6-year-old male cousins began group play therapy after Child Protective Services placed them with their grandmother because each of their parents were abusing drugs. In the first session, one of the boys drew a picture of himself with an angry face kicking the teacher. This was an accurate reflection of his behavior at school, according to his grandmother. The boy's drawing seemed to communicate "I hate," an understandable response to the betrayal he felt due to his mother's abandonment. After about two months of drawing dark and angry pictures, he gradually added color and sunshine. This seemed to reflect the consistent unconditional positive regard he was experiencing in group play therapy and from his grandmother. The next month, he began depicting himself as strong and caring to others through drawings of playing ball with his cousin and giving flowers to his grandmother. His grandmother reported that he had a custodial visit with his mother and said to her "don't do drugs—I love you!" He seemed to have mastered the difference between hating drugs but loving his mother, which released him from consuming anger. After 6 months of group play therapy, his last spontaneous self portrait was a clear indicator of his healing. He drew himself smiling under the sun and simply wrote two powerful words—"I love."

Expressive Arts in Directive or Integrative Group Play Therapy

Preparation.   In directive or integrative group play therapy, the play therapist prepares the play therapy room before children enter by only laying out art materials needed for a specific expressive arts activity. The play therapist must decide if the art activity will take up the entire time or part of the time so that the session can be scheduled accordingly. When it is time to begin the art activity, the play therapist guides children to sit at the table or in a circle on the ground where the art material is set up. The play therapist is advised to begin the session by explaining the parameters of the group art experience so as to reduce any performance anxiety (Chapman & Appleton, 1999).

> "Today, I have prepared art materials for a special activity for each of you to do. Each of your art projects will look different from each other. There is no right way or wrong way to do it. You get to choose how you want to do it."

Ground rules, expectations, and confidentiality are important to communicate to the group to maintain a positive and productive climate.

> "Before I tell you the directions, please remember in here, we work together to make it a safe place for our bodies, art projects, and feelings. Sometimes accidents or mistakes happen and that is O.K. but we will be wise so as not to break things or waste materials on purpose. After we finish the projects, each of you will have a chance to show and talk about your project if you want. Others can say what they

like or find interesting about it. Remember, what others say and do in here is private. You can tell people not here what you did but please do not tell what others said or did in here."

After these guidelines have been discussed and any questions have been answered, the group play therapist will facilitate four stages of (1) motivation; (2) the art activity itself; (3) discussion of the process and product; and (4) closure (Chapman & Appleton, 1999).

Motivation.   Motivation for the activity may begin with a brief statement of the goal for the session. For example, "our goal with this art project is for each of you to learn something about yourself to help you through your parents' divorce." Rubin (2010) recommends evoking expression through warming up activities to help children overcome natural resistances and blocks to creativity. This can be achieved through soft lighting, soothing music, deep breathing, mental imagery, and rhythmic body movements. One visual prompt activity that warms up children is the scribble technique of developing a picture by expanding on a self-made scribble (Winnicott, 1989).

Art Activity.   Given the plethora of expressive art activities that are described in other books (Kaduson & Schaefer, 1997; Malchiodi, 2005, 2008; Rubin, 2010, 2011; Wadeson, 2010), play therapists need to be systematic and deliberate in the chosen activity. Typically, art activities are for "exploration; rapport building; and expression of inner feelings, self-perception, interpersonal relations, or the individual's place in the world" (Rubin, 2010, p. 155). Some suggested art activities for each of these categories are presented in Table 8.1. These activities can be done individually or modified to be done as a group to build cohesion. For example, the activity entitled "self portrait" can be adapted to be "group portrait," while "animal papier mâché" can be modified so that each member adds one part to a "group animal."

For each activity, play therapists can offer children varying degrees of structure or specificity. Media can be pencils, pastels, paints, clay, etc. Themes can be open-ended ("draw what you want") or specific ("draw anger") or symbolic ("draw a witch" to symbolize anger at mother). Implementation can be by each individual or group as a whole. Time length can be limited or unlimited. Method can be typical or novel such as drawing with eyes closed or with the non-dominant hand (Rubin, 2010).

Play therapists are to explain the activity in clear and simple terms and inform participants how many minutes they have for the activity. Time frames help children understand that they do not have to rush so they can pace themselves. While children create, play therapists silently witness the process. The only time play therapists speak during the creation is to remind group members of the ground rules. This reminder is delivered in a soft, friendly but firm voice. Some example explanations and therapeutic responses are provided below.

PLAY THERAPIST: Today, I would like you to draw a picture of yourself. You will have 20 minutes so take some time to think about it and try until you create a picture that you like. Remember, it does not have to be perfect. You can use all the markers

Table 8.1   Group art activities by therapeutic purpose

Category	Suggested Art Activities (Kaduson & Schaefer, 1997; Malchiodi, 2005, 2008; Rubin, 2010, 2011; Sweeney & Homeyer, 1999; Wadeson, 2010)
Exploration	1. "Grab bag creation" using all the materials in a bag (i.e., lump of molding clay, 4 popsicle sticks, 4 pipe cleaners, 4 feathers, 10 beads) to create something. 2. "Left hand versus right hand" simultaneously drawing (or painting) on one large paper with two different colors for the left and the right. 3. "Blindfold drawing" using various markers or crayons to draw something while members are blindfolded. 4. "String in paint" placing string in various paint colors and then pulling it over paper to make different shapes.
Rapport-building	1. "Cooperative group art" with each member choosing one marker color to draw on a 3′ × 6′ piece of paper in silence, with each member using a different color. Then each member uses the same color marker to draw on another large piece of paper, but with permission to talk with other members. 2. "Group scribble" with one member starting the scribble, the next member adding a drawing to make the scribble an identifiable object (e.g., balloon), the next member adding another scribble, the next member adding a drawing to make the scribble an identifiable object out of the scribble (e.g., a cloud), etc. 3. "Group magazine collage" in which each member pastes magazine pictures of five of their favorite things on to one page. 4. "Group three-dimensional creation" in which each member takes turns adding one of their random six items (e.g., popsicle sticks, pipe cleaners, feathers, beads, yarn) to a lump of molding clay.
Expression of inner feelings	1. "Color my feelings" in my body in which members choose different colors to represent different feelings (i.e., black for sadness, red for anger, green for envy, etc.) and coloring in the amount of feelings they feel in different places of their body on a human figure outline (i.e., red in the hands, black on the heart, sadness on the face, etc.). 2. "Bottle out your feelings" in which members wrap water bottles with colored yarn on the outside of the bottle to represent the different feelings they have. Then write a message on paper of what they wish to feel and strategies to manage feelings. Place the message in the bottle. 3. "Mask of outer and inner feelings" in which members draw and decorate the outside of a mask (e.g., paper plate) with the feelings they show people and the inside of a mask with the feelings they keep private or hide from other people. 4. "Bricks for wall and bridges" in which members decorate paper bricks (e.g., tissue boxes) of their inner feelings and stack as a wall around them. Then members knock down one brick at a time to build a bridge to other members.
Self-perception	1. "Self-portrait drawing" in which each member draws self. 2. "Rosebush technique" in which each member draws self as if they were a rose bush.

Category	Suggested Art Activities *(Kaduson & Schaefer, 1997; Malchiodi, 2005, 2008; Rubin, 2010, 2011; Sweeney & Homeyer, 1999; Wadeson, 2010)*
	3. "Animal papier-mâché" in which each member creates and decorates an animal that represents self. 4. "Container sculpture" in which each member uses molding clay to create a container (i.e., cup, pitcher, closed box) that represents the amount of love they can receive and give at this time.
Interpersonal relations	1. "Kinetic family drawing" in which members draw self and each member in their family doing something. "Kinetic school drawing" in which members draw self and members of their classroom doing something. 2. "Three circles of family and friends" in which members draw or visually represent with items people they know in three concentric circles with the inner most circle representing the few people who know them best, the next circle representing people who know them somewhat well, and the outer circle representing people who only casually know them. 3. "Group sculpture" in which members create a three-dimensional object out of clay, wood, paper bag puppets, or popsicle sticks that represents each group member. Then place each object on a surface (upside down shoe box) to show proximity to other family members. 4. Alternatively, "Group mobile" in which members draw or create each family member and/or close friend and hang cut out drawings or objects with yarn on a wire coat hanger that is bent into a circle. 5. "Barrier busters" in which members draw what prevents them from being closer to family and group members and what will bust the barrier so they can get closer.
Individual's place in the world	1. "My community rock garden" in which members find and paint a rock to represent meaningful people and places in their world and arrange it in a shoe box with other objects from nature (leaves, flowers, feathers, etc.). Alternatively, "Community map" in which members draw or build with Legos meaningful people and places in their community. 2. "Coping shield" in which members draw or glue magazine pictures that represent their positive coping strategies and positive family and individual characteristics on a poster board cut in the shape of a shield that is then hung around the neck with yarn. 3. "Friendship bracelet" of different colored beads, representing supportive people, that is strung on yarn or a pipe cleaner. 4. "Star story book" in which members create an autobiography picture book starting with "once upon a time a star was born." Members draw or paste pictures and write text describing significant life events in their own life from the past, present, and future. They represent/describe positive memories from the past, their current challenges, and end their story as an accomplished adult who is then magically transformed into a star in the sky that guides other kids with wisdom and light. Use colored paper, punch holes in the side, and bind with yarn. Decorate the cover page.

and crayons here. I will wait quietly and let you know when you have five minutes left.

ANNABELLE: O.K. That sounds fun. I need a pencil.

PLAY THERAPIST: Annabelle, you are excited. You can find a pencil in the box and start whenever you are ready.

KATELYN: This is stupid. I can't draw good. I'm not doing it!

PLAY THERAPIST: Katelyn, you feel irritated and worried. This is a safe place. You are welcome to try as much as you want and do it however you want. I respect that you each will do it differently.

[Annabelle begins meticulously. Katelyn scribbles for two minutes.]

KATELYN: O.K. I'm done.

ANNABELLE: I'm not done. I just started.

PLAY THERAPIST: We still have 18 minutes for the activity. I'll wait quietly until then. You can choose to draw something else quietly or continue working on your picture of yourself quietly.

ANNABELLE: I'm going to draw a rainbow over mine.

KATELYN: Fine! [Said in an irritated tone.] I'm going to draw mine again with heart balloons. Then I'm going to draw my little ponies.

PLAY THERAPIST: You both have a plan! Continue working quietly.

When children are hesitant or resistant as indicated above, play therapists should maintain unconditional positive regard, empathy, and genuineness while holding firm boundaries in a friendly tone. It is helpful to remember the expressive arts activity and the group is a process. Rubin (2010) identified that members may proceed through different stages in the expressive arts process, specifically through "(1) precursory activities, (2) chaotic discharge, (3) art in the service of defense (stereotypes or copying), (4) pictographs, and (5) formed expression" (p. 150). Thus, play therapists must also be patient as children progress through these stages of art expression.

Discussion of the Process and Product

After the allotted time for creating the art project has ended, the play therapist leads a discussion of the product and process. The play therapist informs the children that they will spend the remainder of the time sharing and discussing their art projects. It is helpful to provide a reminder that the playroom is a safe and respectful environment where one person speaks at a time. The objective of the discussion is not to praise or criticize the art product but to encourage children's self-exploration through the process. Many children will directly ask the play therapist if they like their art project or if it is pretty. A helpful response is "You want me to like it but what is most important is if YOU like it and what you learn about yourself through the art project."

Before inviting a child to speak, play therapists should observe the mood of the art project. Is it empty, lively, disorganized, rigidly organized, chaotic, tranquil, etc.

(Wadeson, 2010)? The mood of an art project can serve as an indicator of the child's current status and progress over time.

Rather than attempting to interpret meaning of the art project, Wadeson (2010) stated therapists should allow the client to state what it means. The play therapist does this by asking the group members "who would like to tell us about their art project first?" Usually children are eager to describe their art and name the people who are represented in it. After the first child has described his or her art project or the group art project, the play therapist can facilitate further discussion with the following statements and open ended questions (Rubin, 2010; Wadeson, 2010):

- "I'm curious about this green shape (or part). Tell us about it."
- "I wonder if you or someone else you know is in here."
- "I notice this one (or part) is close (or far) from this one. Tell us about that."
- "What sort of mood or feeling does your art project have? Sad, lonely, chaotic, happy, etc.?
- "I wonder what this one (or part) is thinking and feeling?"
- "If your creation could talk, what would it say?"
- "Tell me a story about your creation."
- "In this picture, what would happen next?" Or "What would your creation do next?"
- "What is the title of your art project?"
- "What surprised you when you were creating this?"
- When you were creating this, did it remind you of anything or make you think of anything?
- "What did you discover about yourself, family, or others through this process?"
- "What questions, comments, or compliments do the other group members have?"

Rather than asking all these questions, play therapists discern when children have had enough questioning and need quiet reflection. "It is not necessary to plumb any one art expression to its depths. Material in the picture that is significant will emerge repeatedly. The main thing is to encourage the client in her own self-exploration so that this process may continue long after the therapy has ended" (Wadeson, 2010, p. 44).

During the group discussion, play therapists may need to restate or redirect group members' comments about another member's art project to ensure the process is therapeutic. For example, if one group member says "that part is weird," the play therapist can intervene with a restatement of "Vincent, you find that to be different and maybe would like to know more about it. Frida, you were very creative with that part and you can choose to tell us about that part if you want."

After members have shared and processed their art project, play therapists can ask group members if they noticed common themes such as loneliness, strength, loss, hope, etc. Members may also identify common experiences in the process such as enjoyment in being near others while being quiet or getting to know each other in a new way. Identifying common themes and experiences creates a sense of universality and cohesion in the group.

Closure

In the last few minutes of the session, the play therapist leads closure by asking each member to share one thing they learned from the process. Afterwards, the play therapist thanks the group for sharing and reminds the members to maintain confidentiality of what was said and seen during the session. The art projects belong to the creator, not the play therapist. A digital picture of the art project can be taken if children grant permission. It is children's prerogative if they want to take home their own art project or throw it in the trash. If children ask the play therapist to keep the project, then it is treated as part of the clinical record and kept in a locked file cabinet. Play therapists do not display art projects as this would be analogous to displaying client transcripts on the wall (Landreth, 2012).

Conclusion

Art expressions have been used throughout history. Although not everyone is artistic, everyone is creative. Expressive arts are a common modality for play therapists. The rationale for expressive arts includes expression of imagery, decrease of children's defenses, objectification, permanence, spatial relationship, release of creative and physical energy, enhancement of self-esteem, and literature that indicates success.

Play therapists prepare for expressive arts activities by considering group member selection, personal experience with art, physical space, goals, and roles. In nondirective group play therapy, carefully selected expressive art materials are laid out with other toys for children to use when and how they choose. In directive or integrative group play therapy, the play therapist prepares specific art activities and facilitates children through four stages of: (1) motivation, (2) the art activity itself, (3) discussion of the process and product, and (4) closure. Suggested activities for each stage have been provided and a plethora of activities are available.

Play therapists lead a discussion of children's art product and process through a series of open-ended questions. Then, they facilitate closure of the session by asking each member what they learned. Expressive arts in group play therapy allow children to achieve individual and group goals through a safe and creative process. Group play therapists will find motivation by imaging the self-exploration, understanding, and satisfaction that Vincent Van Gogh, Frida Kahlo, and Salvador Dali would have experienced if they were treating them in group play therapy.

Discussion Questions and Learning Activities

1. How would you respond if a parent or school principal asked you "Why should children participate in expressive arts play therapy when they already attend art class at school?"
2. Describe the procedures for selecting clients, materials, and activities for expressive arts group play therapy.
3. Discuss the benefits and limitations of nondirective versus directive expressive arts group play therapy.

4. Demonstrate how you will process the art product with a child who was clearly artistic and created elaborate detail versus a child who was sloppy and created little detail.

5. Plan an 8-week expressive arts curriculum for a group of four 8-year-old boys or population you will be serving.

9   Group Puppet Play

The use of puppets in group play therapy is a valuable therapeutic medium for children to express their perceptions, thoughts, and feelings while maintaining a sense of distance from emotionally threatening material. Puppets provide a fun, spontaneous quality to play that allows children to feel safe in expression. When children use puppets, they are often motivated to engage in interactive play, either between puppets or between puppet and person. Hence, puppet play will often elicit demonstration of internalized processes within the child, as well as social drives and skills.

Puppets have a rich history in child therapy for both diagnostic and therapeutic purposes. Melanie Klein (1929) noted that children used play materials, specifically mentioning puppets, to express the personification of people in their lives, leading to the revelation of sources of anxiety and stages of ego development. Woltmann (1940, 1972) proposed that puppet shows can be used with children to analyze and remedy behavioral problems, specifically asking children to provide solutions to their conflicts and using those solutions as a basis for therapy. Puppet techniques have been used by several researchers to diagnostically assess emotional stability (Irwin, 2000), perceptions (Knell & Beck, 2000; Measelle, Ablow, Cowen, & Cowen, 1998), and family dynamics (Irwin & Malloy, 1994; Ross, 2000) of young children.

Function of Puppets in Group Play Therapy

Bromfield (1995) suggested several functions served by the use of puppets in therapy. Puppets offer a sense of physical and psychological safety in self-expression that allows a child to project conflict and feelings onto puppets without fear of consequences from others. Puppets also allow a child the opportunity to project feelings that may have been unacceptable to the child. The use of puppets is likely to prompt self-revelation on the part of the child. Additionally, children use puppets to play out interpersonal interactions, including physical and verbal aggression that may be unacceptable in reality. Bromfield proposed that the use of puppets was more efficient in prompting disclosure of complicated events more quickly and richly than using verbally inclined therapies. Children may use puppet play to gain mastery over situations in which they feel powerless, as well as reveal their perceptions of events. Puppets have a disinhibiting quality by which the child can be freed for expression while also allowing containment through the holding environment of the puppet itself. Finally, puppets serve the purpose of catharsis, allowing children to work through painful and fearful experiences.

Although puppets have been used in individual play therapy to meet the unique needs of children in emotional expression, they serve more functions in a group environment. Applying a structured play approach to puppet shows, Gendler (1986) concluded that the use of puppets led to six implications regarding the therapeutic functions of puppetry in groups. (1) For younger children, puppets served as transitional objects bridging fantasy and reality; (2) Puppetry provided a means of expression for unconscious needs and fantasies, specifically exposing conflict between these elements. Once children expressed the conflict, puppet play allowed children to work through the struggle, sometimes serving as helpers in the resolution of each other's conflict; (3) Puppet shows provided a safe medium to express feelings that had not been previously expressed; (4) Puppet shows allowed for verbalization of events that could not be spoken of in normal verbal interaction or discussion; (5) Group members used puppet play to relate to each other in an empathic and supportive way; and (6) Production of puppet shows led children to a sense of pleasure and accomplishment, as well as utilized imagination and creativity. Gendler described puppet intervention as "Almost deceptively simple" (p. 52) in its application due to the dynamics provided through projection and group process.

Considerations in Puppet Selection and Use

Whether using puppets in structured or unstructured mediums, a therapist should offer a numerous and diverse collection to children in therapy. The recommended number ranges from a minimum of 15 to 25 puppets, and some therapists would suggest that the number should be higher. Number of puppets available would also depend on the number of group members. If the group number is over five children, the therapist will benefit from having more than a 5 to 1 ratio of puppets to children. Providing ample diversity and number of puppets helps meet the unique needs of each individual child.

Carter and Mason (1998) suggested some basic considerations in selecting puppets. These include choosing puppets that are easy for children to manipulate, do not carry universal fixed symbolism, fit both children and adult hands, are soft and cuddly, are washable or can be dry cleaned. Bromfield (1995) also recommended that puppets with mouths are preferable. Puppets should not have fixed personalities or emotional affect, but should be flexible enough to allow a child to project any personality or emotion (Bromfield, 1995; Carter & Mason, 1998). Puppets should allow for a full range of emotions and actions, including aggressive and nurturing expressions. A diverse collection of puppets includes variations of animals, people, and magical creatures. Puppets are likely to be one of the most expensive materials in a playroom. If a therapist's budget is limited, puppets should be carefully selected and lean toward neutrality. However, many children are attracted to puppets that are colorful, soft, and typically more expensive. Therapists may need considerable time to build up their puppet collection to meet the diverse needs of their client population.

In addition to the selection of puppets, therapists who plan to use puppets in structured or unstructured methods will also consider how a puppet should be handled by the therapist. Carter and Mason (1998) offered additional recommendations on puppetry. In using hand puppets, the therapist should make sure that the puppet is looking at the audience, in this case, group of children. A puppet that is slumping or looking at the floor detracts from the illusion of reality. The therapist should keep the puppet moving in human-like motions throughout use, such as moving hands, legs, or face. The therapist should also move the lower jaw of the puppet when talking, not the upper jaw which is common for inexperienced puppeteers. Emotions on puppets can be manipulated by using the puppeteer's hand to wrinkle the puppet's face. The more a therapist practices, the more realistic a puppet will appear which is likely to encourage children to interact more with the puppet (Carter & Mason, 1998).

Nondirective and Directive Use of Puppets in Group Play Therapy

Nondirective Methods

The purpose of nondirectivity in group play therapy is to allow children to move toward play that is most enhancing for the group, as well as individuals within the group. The therapist's choice to avoid directing children's play is intentional so that children can act with each other as realistically as possible, utilizing their own motivations and skills. Through the therapist's intentional and focused reflections and the safety of the therapist–child relationship, children will become aware of their feelings, needs, and their impact on other children. As a result of self-awareness and self-within-relationships, children will actively work toward more interpersonally effective skills. Hence, the use of puppets in the nondirective playroom is the same as use of any play materials in the playroom. Puppets are one of many types of communication tools for children to speak in their natural language of play (Landreth, 2012). However, the nondirective play therapist will have special considerations regarding puppetry in the playroom.

In a nondirective playroom, a variety of puppets are displayed in the room within reach of the children. Ideally, the play therapist has taken care to ensure that each puppet can be seen and attained easily. Additionally, the playroom includes a puppet theater that is large enough to accommodate three or more children behind it. The puppet theater also has a curtain that can be opened and closed to shield the children and allow them privacy for preparation of puppet choices and stories.

Although the nondirective play therapist may not be directing puppet play, the therapist is still interactive in the play. The children decide whether puppets will be used during play sessions. When a child's puppet addresses the therapist, the therapist responds by making eye contact and responding to the puppet (Bromfield, 1995). If the therapist attempts to talk directly to the child, she has ignored the child's self-direction in play, ultimately devaluing the child's intention. The therapist does not make demands of the puppet or direct the puppet's verbalization, but instead responds to the puppet in the same way she would normally respond to the child. Just as the therapist does not rush the process in play therapy, the therapist does not rush puppet play. The therapist accepts the emotions, thoughts, and actions of the puppet, just as she would the child's emotions and thoughts, only reflecting specific feelings when the affect seems clearly communicated by the puppet. If children use the same puppets in the same manner (e.g., names, personality characteristics, etc.) each session, a therapist may want to remember these details and reflect without prompting from the child in order to communicate her understanding and care for the child's previous sharing. Yet, the therapist should be attuned to the child, allowing the child freedom to change puppet characteristics from session to session, if desired. Finally, Bromfield (1995) warned that the therapist should respect a puppet chosen by the child as an extension of the child, being careful not to inadvertently mistreat the puppet in the child's presence by throwing it into a box or casually tossing it around.

Nondirective Case Example

Adam and Cole were two first-grade boys participating in child-centered group play therapy in a school playroom. Adam was referred because he had been very aggressive with other children. Cole was referred because he was socially awkward and had no friends in school. In their first two sessions, Adam and Cole played in the sand box, taking turns moving vehicles in and out of the box. In the second session, Cole spent a few minutes looking at the puppets, which were displayed in the corner of the room, behind the puppet theater. He never chose or verbalized anything about the puppets. In the third session, the two boys entered the room.

ADAM [to Cole]: I'm going to take the big truck, you take the boat.

THERAPIST: Adam, you've got a plan for today.

COLE [wanders over to puppets, picks up monkey, and looks at therapist]: I like this one.

THERAPIST: Oh, you've chosen a special one for you.

> Adam is intrigued and walks over to the puppets. Adam picks up the dragon puppet and looks at it.

THERAPIST: Adam, it looks like you're checking that one out.

> Cole has now put the monkey on his hand. Adam follows by putting the dragon on his hand.

ADAM [to Cole]: Hey, let's do a show. My dragon is going to eat yours.

> Cole follows Adam behind puppet theater but seems hesitant.

THERAPIST: Cole, you're not so sure about this.

> Adam and Cole whisper behind the theater. The therapist cannot hear what they are saying.

THERAPIST: Seems like you guys are planning.

ADAM [pops up through puppet theater curtain]: Ladies and Gentlemen, today is our show "Big Bad Dragon"

THERAPIST: Oh, it's time for the show. The Big Bad Dragon.

ADAM [dragon appears again and is talking in a rough voice]: I'm the big bad dragon and I'm hungry.

COLE [monkey slightly shows his head and in a light voice]: Hi!

ADAM [as dragon]: I'm going to eat you. Ha! Ha! [Dragon tries to grab the monkey]

COLE [in whiney voice]: No, Mr. Dragon please don't eat me.

THERAPIST [to monkey]: Oh no, you're scared.

ADAM [dragon tries to eat monkey but monkey keeps moving]: C'mon Cole, let me eat you.

COLE [in his own voice]: No, I don't want you to eat monkey, he's special.

THERAPIST: So, monkey is too special to be eaten. But dragon, you're really hungry.

ADAM [in his own voice]: Okay, so let's grab the pig. [Adam grabs the pig puppet and has dragon on one hand and pig on the other]

COLE [as monkey, but he is laughing as he watches dragon eat the pig]: Pig, you better run.

THERAPIST: Monkey, you're safe and Dragon, you got to eat.

ADAM [as dragon]: Yep, and now we're friends. [Dragon walks off with monkey]

In this case, the puppets were used in the CCPT group just as any other playroom material. The children chose themselves to use the puppets. As expected, the children used the puppets to express a conflict that symbolized their social problems at school. In addition, they moved toward a positive resolution of the conflict without direction from the therapist. However, the therapist engaged in the puppet show with both the children and the puppets, alternately reflecting between the two. The therapist attempted to respond to emotions and intentions of children and puppets in order to raise awareness between the children. Both Adam and Cole appeared to have a desire to connect with each other but also wanted their individual needs met. The puppets and puppet show allowed them to express themselves with a sense of distance, providing safety for the enactment of new skills.

Directive Methods

Directive methods in therapeutic puppetry span a lengthy continuum from highly structured to little structure. Highly directive methods in puppetry typically include a therapist who presents a puppet show to a group of children that serves the purpose of teaching an emotion or skill. This type of puppetry in therapy precludes group member interaction and relies on the therapist to direct an educational environment. Lightly structured puppetry may include the therapist asking the children to create their own puppet show but allowing substantial freedom for creativity and interaction. Level of directivity is determined according to treatment goals and theoretical orientation of therapist.

In structured orientations to therapy, such as CBT, the therapist can structure puppetry so that a puppet has the same problem as the child client (Knell & Dasari, 2011). Puppets can then be useful in modeling skills to younger children to learn how to deal with that problem, thereby serving an educational function (Pincus, Chase, Chow, Weiner, & Pian, 2011). In trauma-focused CBT, puppets can be used to engage children and create distance to decrease anxiety and avoidance, encouraging them to reconstruct traumatic events (Briggs, Runyon, & Deblinger, 2011). In these highly structured, educational approaches to therapy, puppets are tools used to present situations to children, gather their perceptions, and teach better skills in dealing with problems within those situations.

Perhaps the most frequent use of puppetry is the less structured method of facilitating puppet plays and puppet interaction to elicit thoughts, feelings, and perceptions of children. The facilitation of puppet plays and interaction generally involves a brief direction from the therapist, creative and free interaction between children, and a processing time facilitated by the therapist. The purpose of these puppet interventions is to help focus a group on a particular topic but then allow children the freedom to move around within the topic to develop better ways of communication and interaction.

Examples of Less-Structured Puppet Interventions

Puppet interview.   Gallo-Lopez (2006) suggested a puppet interview as a method of helping children get to know one another. Each child chooses a puppet and then children within the group interview the puppet using a talk show format. The therapist is the talk show host and children are the audience who take turns asking questions of the puppet to get know the puppet better. This intervention allows for a high level of energy and interaction between group members. The puppets allow distance and provide a vehicle for projection as group members reveal themselves.

Role-play puppetry.   Ludlow and Williams (2006) presented a group model for children whose parents are divorcing. In their model, puppets are used as a primary tool for connecting leaders and children, providing divorce scenarios, eliciting children's thoughts and feelings, and developing coping skills. In the initial session, the therapist uses a family of homemade puppets to present a divorce scenario to children. After the puppet show, the therapist facilitates discussion and reaction to the scenario. Children are then asked to create their own puppets who will be "advisors" to the family. At the beginning of each session, the children use the first 15 minutes of session to create a new puppet to add to their characters. This time serves as an interactive period where group leaders and children connect with one another through sharing. Following interactive time, the therapist facilitates a puppet show and children join the role-play with their puppets. At the end of the play, children are asked to give advice through their puppets. The use of puppets in this intervention allows children to respond to difficult situations that may mirror their own home lives, yet provides distance to develop coping skills to respond to those situations.

Narrative therapy puppetry.   Butler, Guterman, and Rudes (2009) suggested the use of puppets in the context of narrative therapy. Because narrative therapy relies on the client's ability to externalize the problem, puppets are an effective vehicle toward that end. In this intervention, the therapist asks the child to select a puppet that most closely represents the problem for which the child was brought to therapy. The therapist then questions the child on how the puppet represents the problem. These steps allow the client to define and externalize the problem outside of self, key components of narrative therapy. The child may be allowed to keep the puppet and take it home to continue focus on externalization. The therapist helps the child give a voice to the problem by processing and questioning the puppet. The therapist can also engage in helping the child make meaning of events by processing unique outcomes with the puppet, helping the client to see ways in which they have power over the problem.

Therapeutic puppet theater. Carlson-Sabelli (1998) introduced therapeutic puppet theater, an intervention used with hospitalized children with psychiatric problems related to trauma. There are four stages for the sessions: Beginning puppet play, playing with the possibilities, healing metaphors, and processing. In beginning puppet play, the therapist presents a variety of puppets to a small circle of children. The children are asked to select a puppet and introduce their puppets in puppet voice. When being introduced, the therapist or other children may ask what makes the puppet feel safe, what the puppet's favorite place is, and what question would the puppet like all the other puppets to answer. Introductions help the therapist and children understand each other. In the next phase, the therapist announces that it is time for the story, which results in the children negotiating a play using the characters introduced in the beginning phase. As the children negotiate, they are playing with the possibilities of what could happen in the context of problems that were presented. The therapist can ask facilitative questions during this phase to keep children focused and moving toward a direction. This interaction is the theatrical presentation of the puppets. In the third phase, each child, in the character of puppet, presents an ending to the story explored in the middle phase. Endings are not acted out by the group but allow each individual child to choose the direction for his or her puppet. Children are asked to respond to what they liked most or least about the play. The final phase takes place after each session, in which therapists process the session with one another. Processing includes the noticing of themes, interactions, and responses of children, as well as assessment of progress. This theatric intervention provides an opportunity for children to develop both personal and collective meaning, moving their live stories forward (Carlson-Sabelli, 1998).

Facilitated group puppetry. Gendler (1986), Irwin and Malloy (1994), and Bratton and Ray (1999) presented group puppet interventions that were similar in process and procedures. There are four basic steps involved in the intervention: selecting the puppets, planning the show, presenting the show, and processing the experience (Bratton & Ray, 1999). In the first step, the therapist presents a large variety of puppets by either laying them out on the floor or facilitating therapy in a "puppet room" where puppets are displayed. Each child is asked to select one or two puppets and give their puppets a name. Once children have selected a puppet/s, the therapist asks the children to introduce their puppets to the group. In the second step, the therapist asks the children to plan a puppet show that has a story with a beginning, middle, and end. The only rule is that the story cannot be a story they already know from books, television, or movies.

Depending on time in session, the therapist allots a specific amount of time to planning, usually not more than 15 minutes. The therapist also asks the group to title their puppet show. For the third step, the group presents their puppet show to the therapist. Video-recording the session is preferred so that children can watch it later, possibly to facilitate further processing of content or group dynamics. Video-recording also adds to the drama of the intervention, which elevates enthusiasm for the activity. In the fourth step, the therapist facilitates a processing time with the puppets and the children. At the end of the show, the therapist asks the puppets to all appear on stage and then proceeds to ask a few questions of each puppet. Bratton and Ray suggested that during puppet processing, the therapist may be "helping create new interactions between characters, posing questions that assist group members in considering different explanations, challenging belief systems that are portrayed, and reworking the final outcome to a more positive and healthy one" (p. 271). After this processing, the therapist asks the children to come out, sit in a circle, and talk about the puppet show. They are asked to talk about their characters, what they liked or did not like about the process, and if they can apply anything from the show to their real lives.

Directive Case Example

Juliana, Sara, and Isabella were in fourth grade; all three were 9 years old and referred because their parents were divorcing. Two of the girls were referred by their teachers. Juliana had cried several times at school because her parents had been in serious arguments. Sara had become quieter and withdrawn in the last couple of months. Isabella seemed unaffected but her mother referred her because she was worried how the divorce was impacting Isabella.

The therapist decided that a facilitated puppet show would help the girls get to know one another and hopefully provide an opportunity for the girls to express their perceptions of their home situations. After conducting individual play sessions with each of the girls, the therapist brought them together in a group session. The room included a large number of puppets displayed on the floor and a large puppet theater. The therapist asked the girls to pick out one or two puppets and think of a name for their puppets. The therapist then asked the girls to introduce their puppets. Juliana picked a big, floppy-eared dog that she named Floppy, Sara picked a turtle that she named Mac, and Isabella chose a princess who she named Isabella.

The therapist then asked the girls to plan a puppet show with a story that included a beginning, middle, and end, but it could not be a story they had heard before. The therapist asked the girls to let her know when they were ready to present their puppet show. The girls went behind the theater and it appeared that Juliana took charge of planning. Juliana decided that she needed another puppet and asked the therapist if she could get one. The therapist agreed and Juliana ran out to get the large dragon with fire coming from its mouth. After a few more minutes, Juliana yelled: "Ready." The therapist asked the girls to write the title of their show on the front of the puppet theater before they began. Juliana ran out and wrote: "The Night Things Went Dark."

The show started with Floppy walking along and singing, Mac followed behind slowly, and Isabella danced around them. Floppy narrated by saying that it was a beautiful night and everything is safe. The dragon popped up quickly and screamed. Floppy and Isabella both screamed in fear. Mac hid in the corner of the puppet theater. The dragon yelled: "Get out of here, you stupid girls." Floppy begged the dragon not to hurt them. Isabella told Floppy to just smile and the dragon will go away. From the corner,

Mac said: "No, that won't work, you need to be quiet and hide." The dragon began to beat up Floppy, who cried and cried. Isabella announced that she needed to find her prince so she was leaving. Mac disappeared below the theater. Juliana then announced: "The end." The therapist asked the puppets to come up to the top of the theater.

THERAPIST: Wow, that was scary. Mac, you seemed really scared.

SARA: I told them to be quiet.

THERAPIST: You thought they would be safer if they were quieter.

SARA: Yeah, but they didn't listen.

THERAPIST: Isabella and Floppy, why didn't you listen to Mac?

JULIANA: I didn't want to hide.

ISABELLA: I didn't think he would really hurt us.

THERAPIST: So, Floppy you wanted to be out in the open and Isabella, you just thought it would be okay. Dragon, why were you so mad?

JULIANA: Because they were in my home and making noise. And they're stupid.

THERAPIST: You really don't like them.

JULIANA: No, they just needed to go somewhere else.

THERAPIST: You were just trying to protect your space. Floppy, you sure did cry and beg; you seemed really upset.

JULIANA: I just wish he wouldn't yell. I was trying to sing to make him feel better.

ISABELLA: And I was trying to be happy to make him feel better.

THERAPIST: But neither of those things worked. Can you three come out so we can talk a little more?

[The three girls come out from behind the puppet theater and sit in a circle with the therapist. Sara keeps the turtle puppet on her hand. The others are holding theirs.]

THERAPIST: I just thought we could talk about the show. What did you guys think?

JULIANA: We should have fought back. We could have gotten together and killed the dragon.

THERAPIST: You're thinking of some ways to make the ending better.

JULIANA: Yeah, I wish I could make it better.

ISABELLA: Me, too. If you smile a lot, it makes people happy and then they'll be better.

THERAPIST: Isabella, you think that if you can just keep smiling that other people around you will be happier.

ISABELLA: Yeah, it works for my mom. When she's crying, I'll smile and brush her hair and she feels better.

THERAPIST: So, you worry about your mom. You want to be the one who makes her feel better.

JULIANA: There's no way to make my mom happy. She and my dad fight all the time.

THERAPIST: That sounds scary.

JULIANA: It is.

SARA: If everyone would be quieter, they would get along better.

THERAPIST: Sara, if you can just be quiet enough, that'll help the people in your life.

The therapist and girls continued to process the puppet show, moving back and forth between the show and the girls' perceptions of their home lives. The facilitated puppet show allowed the therapist to see the perception of each girl and the coping skills they developed to deal with their current situations. It also allowed them to share with each other to see that they were dealing with similar situations and start to develop a support system for one another.

Conclusion

In the context of group play therapy, puppetry is one vehicle to help children externally communicate their inner worlds and their interpersonal approaches to others. Puppets are unique in the playroom because they encourage children to personify feelings, problems, and people through a safe medium. Additionally, puppets serve as a physical extension of the child, thereby inspiring children to project their most private perceptions. In the group environment, puppets provide enough safety to allow children to experiment with new social and coping skills to improve relationships. Whether used in directive or nondirective settings, puppets are valuable in group play therapy due to children's natural inclination to express themselves through projective means.

10   Group Sandtray Therapy

Another exciting group play therapy intervention is group sandtray therapy, which combines the therapeutic elements of group therapy with the effective expressive intervention of sandtray work.[1] Sandtray therapy is a projective and expressive therapy with compelling flexibility. Sweeney and Homeyer (2009) note: "It can be used with clients of all ages, it can be nondirective and directive, and can be fully nonverbal and projective while also being cognitive and solution-focused" (p. 297).

Homeyer and Sweeney (2011) define sandtray therapy as "an expressive and projective mode of psychotherapy involving the unfolding and processing of intra- and interpersonal issues through the use of specific sandtray materials as a nonverbal medium of communication, led by the client(s) and facilitated by a trained therapist" (p. 4). Fundamentally, it involves the therapeutic use of a collection of miniatures and a container of sand—not unlike art therapy's use of colors and paints on a blank palette.

The tools of the sandtray therapist are basic and simple. First, there are *sand and water*, which are elemental properties of the earth, naturally and kinesthetically appealing. Then there is a *tray*, a container for not only the sand and play media, but also a container of the client's psyche. Finally, there is the *collection of miniatures*, which serves as a universe of symbols and images and more specifically the "words" that clients can present in therapy without having to directly verbalize potentially painful issues. While it is important to note these therapeutic tools, it is more important to emphasize that the sandtray *process* and *product* are the keys that create a milieu in which clients can approach and work through the presenting issues.

There are several types of sandtray therapy groups: individuals working within group settings; same age groups; family groups; parent–child dyads; sibling groups; supervision groups; personal growth groups; professional development experiences. Groups can be found in schools, agencies, private practice, in-service training experiences, and others.

---

1   For readers interested in further exploration on sandtray therapy, consider another Routledge resource: *Sandtray Therapy: A Practical Manual* (Homeyer and Sweeney, 2011).

Brief History of Sandtray Therapy

It is not possible within the scope of this chapter to provide an exhaustive history for the origin of sandtray therapy. A brief glance, however, will provide the new and returning therapist a helpful infrastructure upon which to build.

In the 1920s, following her experience as a physician during the First World War, Margaret Lowenfeld (1979) was looking for a way to connect with her child patients in an honest way, without contaminating the child's communication with adult perceptions, perspectives, or preconceived theories. The traumatic impact of war on the troops, prisoners of war, displaced students, children, and families had a profound influence on Lowenfeld. When she began working with children in the mid-1920s, she explored interventions through which children could communicate their perception of their world. Lowenfeld sought "to find a medium which would in itself be instantly attractive to children and which would give them and the observer a 'language', as it were, through which communication could be easily established" (p. 281).

Lowenfeld remembered a book by H.G. Wells (1911) she'd read, *Floor Games*. In the book Wells shares detailed, lengthy, and involved stories about how he and his sons would play with small toys on the floor of his home. Seeing the application to her work with children, Lowenfeld began collecting miniature toys, and offered children a chance to share their worlds with her in sandtrays. This developing intervention came to be called "The World Technique" (1979).

Others began to employ Lowenfeld's techniques. The primary advancement and promotion of the use of sandtray therapy was Dora Kalff. Kalff was a Jungian-trained therapist, who attended a psychiatric conference where she heard Lowenfeld present her World Technique (Weinrib, 1983). Kalff went to London and studied with Lowenfeld, and returned to her native Switzerland, developed a distinctively Jungian approach to sandtray therapy, which she termed "Sandplay" (Kalff, 1980). Kalff had been strongly influenced by Jung's mentoring and her experience with Eastern mysticism while living in the Far East.

An important distinction needs to be made here. The term *sandplay* is often used to describe any psychotherapeutic use of the sandtray and miniatures. The term sandplay, however, specifically applies to the Jungian approach to sandtray therapy. While the approaches of Lowenfeld and Kalff remain the primary approaches to the therapeutic use of the sandtray, there are other orientations that have been developed over the past several decades.

General Process of Sandtray Therapy

Before discussing group sandtray therapy, it is important to provide background on the general process of sandtray. This includes the basic materials required and a simple process. Homeyer and Sweeney (2011) discuss an eclectic approach to sandtray therapy, recognizing that therapists bring a wide variety of theoretical and technical perspectives.

The materials used in sandtray therapy can be entirely basic or exceptionally elaborate and detailed. It is absolutely not imperative, however, to invest a great deal of expense or even office space in the development of an adequate collection of sandtray miniatures. An elaborate set-up may in fact be overwhelming for either individual or group clients, and may arguably serve to meet the needs of group play therapists more than their clients. It is helpful for sandtray therapists to receive supervision and consultation about their media selection as much as the sandtray process itself. The basic materials needed include the sandtrays and a selection of miniatures.

Commonly, the sandtrays used in individual sandtray therapy are themselves 20″ × 30″ × 3″, and are painted blue on the inside to simulate sky and water. Depending on the size of the group being worked with, this size may or may not be adequate. Adaptations on size and number of trays will be discussed below.

The size of the tray is important, as it naturally provides boundaries and limits for clients. Also, it is helpful if the sandtray session creation can be viewed in a single glance. This may not be possible if using a larger tray for group sandtray. Trays should be waterproof, so that they can be used for both wet and dry sand. The tray(s) should be set on a stable surface, preferably at about average desk height, with room around the base of the tray. Some clients like to position miniatures *outside* of the tray, perhaps representing intrapsychic or interpersonal issues that are not ready to be fully approached and processed in the tray. Also, it may be helpful to store tray(s) on a mobile cart that can be moved from the corner of the therapy room to the middle so clients can work with it. It is helpful for clients to be able to access trays from all sides.

Trays should be filled—one third to one half—with quality sand. Although inexpensive, it may not be best to use playground sand, which often contains small pebbles, or sand that is too fine, which can result in powder and cause allergic reactions. There are various colors and textures of sand available. Also, alternative materials are used, such as rice, which is certainly easier for cleaning up if spilled. We strongly prefer sand, as the kinesthetic and sensory qualities seem to impact clients at a deeper level.

A selection of miniatures should be made available for use in the sandtray. It is generally suggested that miniatures be 2–3″ in height. Unlike a collection of miniatures for hobby purposes, however, the issues of scale and proportion are not a concern. In fact, Homeyer and Sweeney (2011) suggest having predatory animals that are purposively part of a sandtray collection that are disproportionate large, as they may represent the inordinate power differential between victims and perpetrators. Like toys in play therapy, sandtray miniatures should be selected exclusively for the sandtray therapy process—not collected.

Thousands of miniatures are not necessary (and may in fact be emotionally flooding for some clients), but it is helpful to offer a wide assortment of toys and objects. Sweeney (2011b) suggests 300–400 for individual sandtray therapy. It is arguable that having double this for group sandtray would be appropriate. Some basic categories include the following:

- Buildings (houses, castles, factories, schools, churches, stores)
- People (various racial/ethnic groups, military, cowboys, sports figures, fantasy, mythological, various occupations)
- Vehicles (cars, trucks, planes, boats, emergency vehicles, farm equipment, military vehicles)
- Animals (domestic, farm, zoo, wild, marine, prehistoric)

- Vegetation (trees, shrubs, plants)
- Deities (both western and eastern religions)
- Structures (fences, bridges, gates, highway signs)
- Natural objects (rocks, shells, driftwood, feathers)
- Miscellaneous (jewelry, wishing well, treasure chest)

Sensitivity to issues of diversity should always be considered in the selection of miniatures. Fundamentally, it is important to have miniature people (of both genders) reflecting a variety of ethnocultural groups. For example, the use of sandtray therapy in a predominately Latino community with a miniature collection containing only Caucasian figures would be essentially inappropriate. Another example of diversity would be geographical sensitivity and consistency—for example, it is better to have miniature pine trees when working in the forest town and cactuses when working in a desert community.

It is important that miniatures be grouped together by category, and preferably displayed on open shelves. Other manners of display and presentation are possible, but sandtray clients are simply less likely to rummage through bin containers or drawers than they are to select objects from a shelf. Therapists should also consider how to display the miniatures, as the emotionally fragile client is less likely to select a bunny at the feet of a fire-breathing dragon. Also, in the same way impatient or reticent clients may not rummage through a bin, they could also be less willing to search through a disorganized shelf. Therapy offices used for several purposes may necessitate a covered bookcase to hold miniatures, so they will not be a distraction when not in use.

Homeyer and Sweeney (2011) describe six phases of the sandtray therapy process: (1) preparation of the sandtray setting; (2) introduction of the process to the client; (3) creation of the sandtray; (4) post-creation phase; (5) sandtray cleanup; and (6) documentation of the session. Issues specific to group sandtray therapy will be discussed further below. These six phases are briefly summarized:

1. Preparation of the sandtray setting is simple but imperative. The therapist should ensure that the sandtray(s) and miniatures are in place. This includes verifying that no miniatures are buried in the sand from previous sessions and ensuring that the sand is relatively flat and smooth. The room arrangement should provide easy access to the materials, and the therapist should sit in a nonintrusive place.
2. The introduction of the sandtray process can be directed or nondirected, depending on the therapeutic intent. The client can be invited to create a "world" (or scene/picture) in the tray using any number of miniatures, or can be directed to make a specific scene around an event or emotion in the client's life or on a general or specific theme.
3. The creation of the tray, especially in the early stages of sandtray therapy, is often left entirely up to clients. The therapist may make few or no verbalizations to clients and provide complete nonverbal attendance to the clients' work. The therapist may choose to ask questions about the scene as it is unfolding. Some sandtray therapists prefer to let the creative process stand alone, which may be the therapist's judgment, or a reflection of the theoretical orientation to sandtray

therapy. While this may be valuable, we believe that the process needs to be conversational and interactive. Thus, the creation frequently serves as a springboard for discussion with the client.

4. The post-creation phase is a primary aspect of the sandtray therapy process. It is most often appropriate and even necessary to discuss the tray with clients. Generally, clients are asked to give a title to the tray and, as with narrative approaches to therapy, tell their story—the sandtray process provides a projective and expressive means to do this. Clients can be asked to describe the whole scene or portions of it, or to discuss specific miniatures. They may be asked if they are themselves represented in the tray, if other specific persons are in the tray, and are often asked what miniature(s) in the tray have the greatest power.

   If the tray seems like an ongoing scene, clients can be asked about what happened previously or what would happen if the scene were to continue. It may be helpful to frame the process as a client making a movie, and the tray represents the pause button being pushed during an action sequence. This creates the opportunity to discuss future and preceding events, or allows the tray to stand with minimal discussion.

   It is important for sandtray therapists to consider several things in the evaluation of client sandtrays. This includes an evaluation of the creation process itself, the sandtrays' contents, the clients' stories, and the therapist's own affective response to the tray. We would emphasize a caution against being too interpretive, stressing the importance of the clients' own interpretation of the therapeutic metaphors in their own creation.

5. The sandtray cleanup may be done as a part of the session or after the client has left. Since the tray represents an expression of the client's own emotional and relational world, therapists are advised *not* to clean that world up without the client's direction and approval. It might be unfair to ask clients to "clean up" their own worlds, as this might communicate that their emotional expression is unacceptable in some way. It can be helpful to remind clients that others use the tray and miniatures, thus their tray cannot be preserved until the next session.

6. Documentation of the session should include routine client progress notes, but should also include a photograph or sketch of the client's tray. This provides a visual and chronological record of the therapy process, which can be shared with clients to facilitate discussion and progress review. Homeyer and Sweeney (2011) include sandtray therapy session chart formats in their text.

While the materials and process are important, it is the role of the sandtray therapist that is the key element. The sandtray therapist is a fellow sojourner with the sandtray client(s), and a facilitator of an interactive and relational process. Hunter (2006) summarizes this well: "The therapist is both the witness, attending with mindful awareness, silent attention, and nonjudgmental presence at each moment, and the participant-observer, attempting to see from the child's perspective, build the relationship, convey caring and encouragement, and facilitate decision making" (p. 279).

Sandtray Therapy with Groups

As with any group play therapy experience, it is important when developing a sandtray therapy group experience to clearly identify the purpose of the group. This will guide the process of the group sandtray experience, as well as the selection of group members.

There are some important factors to remember when putting together a sandtray group. As always, it is crucial to remember developmental age. If you are working with very young children, it is best to keep the total group numbers small—two or three is appropriate. The group sandtray experience may well be similar to holding concurrent sessions, as young children normally alternate between individual and cooperative play. They will frequently weave back and forth between these types of play, and at times it will seem like the therapist is holding two or three separate sandtray therapy sessions that just happen to be occurring in the same room at the same time. Also, with younger children, mixing genders in the group is quite appropriate.

This is mentioned because for groups made up of older children, single gender groups may be most appropriate. This can remove the developing dynamics of sexual issues, which can complicate group member interactions during the sessions. This will be a clinical judgment call, as sandtray groups focused on a particular presenting issue may be more important than blending or separating by gender.

Sandtray therapy group size will often need to be limited by the available sandtray therapy equipment—size and/or number of sandtrays and number of available miniatures. As always, the therapist's ability to appropriately and therapeutically attend to all sandtray group members is the most important issue when it comes to group size.

Setting Up the Sandtray Group Space

It is important that there is adequate space in the group sandtray setting to allow physical movement of group members around the sandtray, as well as access to and from the miniature collection. As noted earlier, the miniature collection needs to be well organized. While the number of miniatures for a group sandtray experience must be larger for a group, it does not have to consist of thousands. It is hard to arrive at the "right" number, and we are reticent to make a suggestion. However, for a sandtray group of 4–6 members, a sufficiently adequate collection would be around 1,000 miniatures. Recognizing that many sandtray and sandplay therapists have more than this for individual clients, however, we would simply say that this is an individual clinical decision.

Having said this, remember that just as an expansive collection can be overwhelming for an individual client, it can also be for a sandtray group. Homeyer and Sweeney (2011) comment:

> The collection, however, does not need to be, say, for a group of four people, four times the size of a typical collection. The collection does not need to have four of each item. A benefit of the group process is learning how to share and manage limited resources. However, because we also believe that the miniatures are the client's words, symbols, and are used to develop metaphors, we also need to have a sufficient number and variety of miniatures so group members can express themselves.

(p. 64)

The sandtrays can also come in various shapes and sizes. If group members will be doing parallel individual trays, it is obviously best to have same-sized trays for each group member. While the "standard" tray for sandtray therapy is generally 20″ × 30″ × 3″, it is not necessary to have several of this size. It would not be appropriate for one or two of the group members to have this size, while others have smaller trays. For the sake of being egalitarian and avoiding an appearance of favoritism, each group member should have the same size tray.

In terms of office space, it is often difficult to provide each group member with the "standard" size tray. It is suggested that each person be provided a smaller tray, perhaps 10″ × 10″ in size. This general size can be square, rectangular, oval, octagonal, or another shape, depending on the preference of the therapist. The material of the tray (e.g., wood, plastic, etc.) can vary. For the sake of minimizing expense, the take-home plastic food trays from restaurants can be used.

Obviously, a communal group tray must be larger. It is possible to use the standard 20″ × 30″ × 3″ tray for a group, but we would suggest that the group be no larger than four members. Even this size may be limiting, however.

It is not difficult to construct a larger tray, even one that can easily be transported and stored. Homeyer and Sweeney (2011) provide simple instructions:

> Everything can be found at a home center store, and no carpentry skills are needed. Ask for two six-foot-long, 1-inch by 4-inch pieces of wood to be cut in half. These will serve as the four sides of the sandtray. Use corner braces (found in the carpentry section of the store) to hold the four pieces of wood together … Drape a blue painter's cloth inside the wooden sides and fill with two bags of play sand. Voila! You have a three-foot-square group sandtray. This size will easily accommodate 5–7 people …. Also available at home centers stores are 5-gallon buckets. Store the sand, the blue cloth, and corner brackets in these buckets until needed again.
>
> (p. 64)

Group sandtray therapists may choose to temporarily divide the larger group sandtray into "individual" sections. This can be advantageous when doing therapeutic work with enmeshed or disengaged groups (or families), as well as when shifting to and/or from doing group trays to individual trays. This can be accomplished by providing artificial "walls," preferably made from solid material such as wood or plastic. We have found that simply drawing lines in the sand or using something like cardboard tends to be fragile and insubstantial, perhaps reflecting the unclear or inappropriate boundaries in group members' relationships.

These dividers can create as many quadrants in the larger tray as may be necessary. Group members may initially have their own "section" in which to work, while simultaneously having at least visual access to (and thus participating with) the larger family tray. If it becomes appropriate, and is therapeutically intentional, the dividers can be removed or reconfigured, for the group to work on issues within subsystems or as a collective group.

If doing group sandtray therapy with preschoolers, it is usually helpful to have deep trays, whether individual trays or a larger group tray. The simple truth is that young children are considerably active, and will often place and move miniatures in the tray—as if it were a play therapy experience, in miniature. Sand often flies around, not necessarily intentionally but simply as a part of the play process. We would argue that it would not be appropriate to set limits here, as the spilling of the sand comes from normal, age-appropriate movement. Thus, the deeper trays can help both therapists and group members by naturally limiting the distraction of accidental sand spills.

After the collection of miniatures and sandtrays, the important third material needed is the sand. While other materials are occasionally used, we strongly prefer sand, because of its sensory and kinesthetic quality. It is important that the sand is hygienic, and not too fine (when it can be powdery and cause allergic responses) or too coarse (when it can contain irritating small pebbles). Different colors and textures are available, and often vary according to the preference of the therapist. It is possible to use miniatures on a flat surface—such as when constructing genograms using sandtray miniatures to represent family members—but the mere sensory manipulation of the sand has therapeutic value.

Working with Individuals in a Sandtray Group Setting

As noted above in the discussion of sandtrays, one valuable format for group counseling is having individual group members create their own individual sandtrays in the context of the group setting. This is fundamentally a form of parallel play. The entire group therapy experience may consist of this format, or it may be used as an introduction to a group sandtray, or to shift back and forth from parallel individual trays to a shared group process. Kestly (2010) discusses a group process of individual work within a group, which she calls sandtray friendship groups. Kestly recommends groups of 2–6 or more, noting that groups with higher numbers of children generally require more than one group facilitator. When group members are ready to shift from the individual trays to the large group or "communal" tray, Kestly recommends that the large group tray be on the floor and 4′–5′ in diameter or square (if working with a larger group of children). She recommends 10–12 weekly sessions, of about one hour in length. Younger children may find 45 minutes adequate. We have found even a half-hour session is often adequate.

A typical hour-long session allows for 30–40 minutes of building time with a 5-minute warning when the allotted building time is about completed. The remaining 15–20 minutes is used for group members sharing the stories of their trays. Kestly (2010) reminds us that young children often find it challenging to stay quiet while others are telling their tray stories. The therapist needs to be sensitive to this age-appropriate situation, and may choose to allow young children to play quietly in their trays while others are talking. Therapists often need to assist children, by therapeutically prompting them to share their stories and keeping other children attentive and nonintrusive.

This same dynamic may well be true when adapting this intervention with adolescents and adults. Therapists can encourage older group members to be "tour guides," a term that would be more developmentally appropriate, as they lead other group members through the world they have created. This is an empowering dynamic for all group members.

De Domenico (1999) also discusses the behavior of children working individually in a group sandtray setting. This again applies to clients of all ages. She notes that as group members look at each other's trays, they have the opportunity to show respect for the other group members' worlds. Group members enjoy "visiting" each other's worlds, and will often comment on each other's ingenuity in the creation of their trays. They also can help solve each other's building dilemmas and are eager to hear others' stories. As all therapeutic groups' experiences facilitate, group members are able to work out on their own a new way to interact with each other.

Considering Yalom's (2005) group therapeutic factors, individual group members note both similarities and differences in their sandtray creations. This universality is an important dynamic in meaning as applied to miniature selection and placement. As group members visit each other's trays, there may be an amount of copying or "contamination" will occur from one builder to another. For example, Homeyer and Sweeney (2011) note "in one 5th grade boys group, one boy placed a small blue foam container/box (it once held fruit) into the sand and filled it with water. It subsequently appeared in all the other boy's trays" (p. 66).

The universal learning that one is not alone that should occur in all group therapy experiences certainly occurs in group sandtray therapy. This key therapeutic dynamic counters the common factor of isolation and secrecy that can so often bind the emotional lives of individual and group clients. The benefit of group therapy is that it removes the sense of being "different" that group members bring into the group experience. Sandtray groups carry an ability to develop insight into self and others' experiences. An important dynamic that can eventuate is a toleration of different viewpoints—beginning with a toleration of other group members' sandtray worlds—which is critical for the development of empathy and respect of others.

Shifting from advanced individual work to a communal sandtray requires more trust, patience, faith, interest in one another, and tolerance of others' attitudes and behaviors (De Domenico, 1999). This shift leads to the development of a group ego, as members begin to understand the impact of their own action on others.

Group Sandtray Experiences

The exciting thing about both individual and group sandtray therapy is its adaptability. Almost every group play therapy intervention discussed in other chapters in this book can be adapted for use in the sandtray. Sandtray miniatures can take the role of puppets (Chapter 9). The sandtray and miniatures can serve as substitutes for most expressive arts interventions (Chapter 8). Sandtray therapy can be used in schools (Chapter 13) and can be used for bereavement and loss issues (Chapter 14). Using a portable set up—miniatures arranged by category, placed in small boxes, and put in a rolling suitcase, together with a smaller plastic sandtray—sandtray therapy can be used for crisis work (Chapter 12). Most of the directive and prescriptive interventions discussed in Chapter 7 can be adapted to the sandtray process. Group sandtray therapy is amazingly versatile and malleable!

Sweeney (2011b), Sweeney and Homeyer (2009), and Homeyer and Sweeney (2011) suggest several cognitive-behavioral applications to sandtray therapy that can be adapted for group experiences. Using the solution-focused "miracle question" (de Shazer, 1988), group members can be asked: "If you woke up tomorrow, and sometime during the night a miracle happened and the problem that brought you here today was solved just like that, I wonder what that might look like? Could you make a sandtray of this? I wonder what your tray would be like, knowing this had happened?" (Homeyer & Sweeney, 2011, p. 59).

There are other solution-focused questions (de Shazer & Yolan, 2007) that can be adapted for group sandtray use. These can be asked when doing parallel individual sandtrays in a group setting, or the group can be asked to come up with a collective answer. Again, rather than asking for a verbal response, therapists can ask group members to create sandtrays that illustrate the answers. Homeyer and Sweeney (2011) suggest possibilities:

- Could you make a tray that shows when was the last time this was not a problem?
- This challenge could be a lot bigger—could you make a tray about how you've kept this from getting to be a bigger problem?
- If someone were making a movie about you, having resolved this problem, could you make a tray of what hitting the pause button on this movie would look like?
- Can you make a tray showing what you see down the road for yourself after this is resolved?
- How will you even know that this is resolved? Can you make a tray on what this looks like?
- This past week—when you chose not to [argue, get depressed, act out]—what was it like? Can you make a tray about this?
- This past week—when you chose to [argue, get depressed, act out]—what was it like? Could you make a tray about how you'd like to do it differently?
- Can you make a tray on what you might be doing, if you were to "act as if" there was no problem? What would it look like?
- When you were dealing with this challenge a little better than you are right now, what did that look like? Could you make a tray of that? Could you make a tray on what you might need to do in order to get back there?
- If someone threw you a victory parade after you've journeyed though this, could you make a tray on what the parade would be like?
- If your partner/friend/family member were here and making a tray about you, what would it look like? Can you make this tray?
- If I were making a sandtray to describe you—what kind of a tray would I make about you? Can you make this one?
- If you picked a miniature to represent you and another to represent the challenge that brought you into counseling, what would these be? If you picked one or more miniatures to represent what it would take to subdue the one you chose to represent the challenge, what would these be?
- When things are moving in the right direction, what will that look like? Can you make a tray on this? Who will be the first to notice? What miniature would you select for this person?

- Can you make a tray on what is happening right now that you'd like to continue happening? What might you add to the tray to make this happen more?

(p. 59)

Most, if not all, of Beck's cognitive distortions—such as overgeneralization, minimization, dichotomous thinking, arbitrary inference, etc. (Beck & Weishaar, 2005)—can be challenged in the group sandtray therapy process. Again, whether individually or as a group, Homeyer and Sweeney (2011) give an example:

> *Selective abstraction*, defined as "conceptualizing a situation on the basis of a detail taken out of context, ignoring other information" (Beck & Weishaar, 2005, p. 247). This might emerge in the sandtray with the client who becomes suspicious of a colleague who gets a promotion because her office location is closer to the supervisor's: "It must be frustrating not to get this promotion that you were expecting. It's hard to say how much office location played into the decision, but since you don't have control over that, I wonder if you could make a tray about several things you could change in your work that could help for the next promotion cycle." This could help clients focus on what they do have control over, as well as explore other possibilities for the missed opportunity.

(p. 61)

Other techniques that can be used with sandtray groups include: (1) role-playing, using the miniatures; (2) family and school genograms, with miniatures representing group members, family members, friends, and school personnel; (3) issue-focused sandtrays, such as divorce, blended families, school problems, chronic illness, grief and loss, abuse recovery, etc.; (4) clinical supervision; (5) individual, collective, and mutual storytelling—using miniatures as characters; (6) psycho-educational group work; (7) structured rituals; and (8) enactment and reenactment. These are some we have used. This list can certainly go on.

Group Phases

In her chapter on "Group Sandtray-Worldplay", De Domenico (1999) identifies several phases of group sandtray therapy. These are similar to phases and stages in group process in general. The initial, or early phase, finds members are tense, apprehensive, and anxious. They tend to be territorial and possessive. We know that this is a time when group members are looking to see how they fit in, whether or not it is safe to share, and what group rules must be followed. The fundamental role of the therapist according to De Domenico is that of being a witness, to reflect the process, and not to interpret. As sharing within the group occurs, safety grows, resulting in more genuine responses. Empathy and curiosity should increase. Group members learn how to claim their own space as well as consider their contribution to the group process and the created sandtrays. Group members discover their own unique impact on the group and the world as they explore concepts of personal and social responsibility. For sandtray groups where members are working within the same tray, people working in their own space generally mark this stage. Little, if any, relationship between the creations exists. Group members tend to do their own building without paying any attention to the building of others.

As the therapy process continues, group cohesion begins to take shape. Seeing the sandtray group members' issues surrounding rejection, exclusion, inclusion, and need for support marks this second stage. There is an increasing sense of belonging as members become more aware of the group vision for "world" being created. Group acceptance increases, and the involvement in the development of group ideas increases. This will show in the tray as individuals still work in their own area of the tray (De Domenico, 1999). However, group members begin to discuss what they each are creating and will begin to add secondary items to the tray, to in some artificial way bridge or connect the individual creations. If the group tells the story of the group tray, the story tends to be very disjointed, although linked in some way. We will also see that personal issues are evident in the sandtray, often before the group member is prepared to be aware of it and/or can talk about it.

Stage 3 is marked by individuals still selecting miniatures, but then discussing the emerging story with group members before and/or during placement in the sandtray. As the creation or story unfolds, more miniatures are added which demonstrate increased cohesiveness to the story. This is what De Domenico (1999) says is typically labeled as the working stage. Directed prompts from the therapist can be valuable at this stage, to help focus the group on specific therapeutic issues.

Stage 4 is identified when group members have an evident sense of a self-created community (De Domenico, 1999). It can be identified as the development of relationships and increased cooperation. Group members often display their excitement regarding the synergy of their group and the group tray creations. The creation and building process will now frequently involve some level of discussion as they select their miniatures. The cohesion of the selected miniatures and sandtray creation stories greatly increases.

Finally, Stage 5 is identified by an integrated story. Group members will now discuss what they plan to build in the tray before the selection of miniatures. The creation in the tray is created with the plan discussed in mind, although there may continue to be modifications or changes to the story (De Domenico, 1999). The creations now are clearly relational and community-based.

Conclusion

Group sandtray therapy is, like many interventions in this book, an exciting intervention that can bridge theoretical approaches and incorporate a wide variety of technical applications. The sensory and kinesthetic nature of sandtray therapy increases its value as a group play therapy intervention. Adolescents and adults, who may be turned off by the term "play therapy", are often amenable to using sandtrays, as opposed to other interventions that may seem too childish. Sandtray therapy crosses developmental lines as easily as it crosses theoretical approaches.

11　Activity Group Therapy for Adolescents

Adolescence is a new birth, for the higher and more completely human traits are now born. … new qualities of body and soul now emerge … suggestive of some ancient period of storm and stress when old moorings were broken and a higher level attained … Passions and desires spring into vigorous life, but with them normally comes the evolution of higher powers of control and inhibition.

(Hall, 1904, p.xii)

Hall (1904), known as "the father of adolescents," stated that adolescence is a period of "storm and stress" (Arnett, 1999). Hall also believed that organized play was central in making adolescents moral and strong. In light of recent cognitive and neuroscience findings, Hall's propositions have been reconsidered (Arnett, 1999; Casey et al., 2010; Dahl & Hariri, 2005). New research suggests that the "storm and stress" model should not be over generalized to all adolescents, but rather viewed in light of a complex interaction between rising levels of hormones, brain development, genetics, environmental factors, and social context that impacts each adolescent in unique ways (Casey et al., 2010; Dahl & Hariri, 2005). Although "storm and stress" is more likely during adolescence than other developmental periods, the potential for exuberant growth, satisfaction, and resilience can be just as strong (Arnett, 1999; Casey et al., 2010). In fact, scientists have recently conceptualized "the neural plasticity of puberty as a 'finishing school' for social behaviors" (Dahl & Hariri, 2005, p. 373). Therefore, rather than over-emphasizing "storm and stress" of adolescents, I (Baggerly) propose that adolescence may be more accurately described as a period in which adolescents are "seeking sensations to soar."

This positive reframe can be a motivator for play therapists to offer Activity Group Therapy (AGT) for adolescents. Over half a century ago, Slavson (1944) recommended activity-based treatment to meet the developmental needs of troubled youth. Yet, the typical play therapy approaches that play therapists implement with younger children may be viewed as juvenile for adolescents (Ginott, 1961). Therefore, play therapists need to know how to form and implement procedures for AGT that adolescents will enjoy. The purpose of this chapter is to (a) revisit adolescent development in light of new scientific findings, (b) discuss the definition and rationale for AGT, and (c) explain AGT preparation and procedures.

Adolescent Development Revisited

Based on the explosion of scientific research in the past decade, it is prudent to revisit adolescent development from five vectors of (a) physical and neurophysiology, (b) cognitive, (c) emotional, (d) behavioral, and (e) social. Understanding adolescents' developmental needs will guide play therapists in identifying appropriate treatment goals and stimulating strategies.

Physical and Neurophysiology

The physical hallmark of adolescence is puberty. Adolescence begins with the onset of puberty as testosterone in males and estrogen in females stimulate the growth of primary and secondary sexual characteristics (Berk, 2010). In males, pubertal changes include growth of testes from ages 9½ to 13½, growth of pubic hair from 10 to 15, growth spurt from 10½ to 16, change in voice from 11 to 15, spermarche from 12 to 14, and acne from 12 to 17 (Berk, 2010). Females experience an earlier onset of pubertal changes with growth of pubic hair from ages 8 to 14, growth of breasts from 8 to 13, growth spurt from 9½ to 14½, menarche from 10 to 16½, underarm hair from 10 to 16, and acne from 10 to 16. The onset of puberty is influenced by individual variables such as heredity, nutrition, ethnicity, and exercise. Growth spurts in adolescence increase rapidly over four years with gaining approximately 10 inches in height and about 40 pounds. This growth spurt results in ravenous eating in adolescence, yet typically adolescents get unhealthy food. Body and facial parts experience asymmetrical growth, resulting in awkward appearance and movement.

The consequences of the timing of puberty differ based on gender (Berk, 2010). For girls, early maturing tends to result in being unpopular and withdrawn as well as having low confidence, more deviant behavior, and a negative body image (Berk, 2010). In contrast, late maturing in girls results in being popular, sociable, lively, and having a positive body image. For boys, the reverse is experienced. Early maturing in boys results in being popular, confident, independent, and having a positive body image. However, late maturing in boys tends to result in being unpopular, anxious, talkative, attention-seeking, and having a negative body image (Berk, 2010). This difference in reaction of puberty is based on desirable social norms in the United States for girls to be thinner and smaller and boys to be bigger.

Other biological factors impacting adolescent development include changing sleep patterns. A biological-based shift in circadian preferences occurs so that adolescents prefer to go to bed later and sleep in longer in the morning, although it can be controlled by limiting bright artificial light and arousing activities (Dahl & Hariri, 2005). Sleep researchers have determined that 8¾ hours of sleep are optimal for adolescents. Yet, early wake-up times for school and late-night activities result in most teenagers being sleep-deprived.

The neurophysiological hallmark of adolescence is the dominance of the amygdale over the prefrontal cortical region. Brain development during adolescence entails numerous structural and functional changes, especially in the prefrontal cortical region and amygdale. There is extensive growth, pruning of unused synapses, and myelination (i.e., connectivity of different regions of the brain) in the frontal lobe (executive functioning of planning, reasoning, and judgment), parietal lobes (information integration), temporal lobes (language and emotional regulation), and corpus callosum (integrating hemispheres) (Berk, 2010). Yet, an imbalance in the development of subcortical limbic (e.g., amygdale) relative to the prefrontal cortical regions that control reasoning cause intense and frequent negative affect during early adolescent years (Casey et al., 2010). The dominance of the amygdale over the prefrontal cortical regions also results in adolescents having impaired judgment, lack of insight, and proneness to risk-taking behavior (Bunge, 2009). In fact, the brain does not become fully developed with prefrontal cortex dominating most behavior until the mid twenties.

Cognitive

The cognitive hallmark of adolescence is abstract thought. The change from concrete to formal operational thinking begins around the age of 11 and fully develops between the ages of 15 and 20 (Piaget, 1962). Formal operational thinking allows adolescents to engage in abstract thinking and hypothesis testing, specifically being able to deduce hypotheses from a general theory and evaluate the logic of verbal propositions (Inhelder et al., 1958). Numerous aspects of information processing improve in adolescence, such as attention, inhibition, metacognition, cognitive self-regulation, speed of thinking, and open-mindedness (Berk, 2010). Negative consequences of abstract thought include extreme self-consciousness, sensitivity to criticism, idealism, and feeling overwhelmed in planning and decision-making due to inexperience (Berk, 2010).

With the development of abstract thought, adolescents embark on their journey as a philosopher (Kohlberg & Gilligan, 1972). They begin questioning societal conventions as they search for a new self, differentiated from the previously held assumptions. Therefore, adolescents seek cognitive stimulation. Their questioning and desire for discussion must be taken seriously for the successful resolution of identity formation.

Emotional

The emotional hallmark of adolescence is moodiness. Due to the dominance of the amygdale combined with surging hormones, extreme variations in mood from despair to elation to anger and back to elation can occur throughout the day and week. Emotional outbursts, particularly of anger, are common. Depression is also common, affecting 15–20% of adolescence and twice as many girls as boys (Berk, 2010). Arnett (1999) reports "adolescents do indeed report greater extremes of mood and more frequent changes of mood, compared with preadolescents or adults. Also, a number of large longitudinal studies concur that negative affect increases in the transition from preadolescence to adolescence" (p. 320). As a result, conflict frequency between adolescents and parents is highest in early adolescence and conflict intensity is highest in mid-adolescence (Arnett, 1999).

Erikson (1963) described the social-emotional task of adolescents as identity versus role confusion. If adolescents successfully resolve this task of developing an identity, they will be able to define who they are; a direction in life; and commit to vocation, personal relationships, ethnic groups, and ideals. In contrast, if they remain in role confusion, they will have lack of direction and definition of self, restricted exploration, and be unprepared for adulthood. During this social emotional task of developing an identity, adolescents frequently experience identity crises, which are temporary periods of seeking experience and experimenting with different alternatives before determining their own set of values, beliefs, and goals. As new dimensions of self are discovered, adolescents unify and organize traits into a self identity. High self-esteem occurs through high levels of exploration, meaningful activities, and commitment to values (Berk, 2010).

Behavioral

The behavioral hallmark of adolescence is risky behavior. Arnett (1999) reported "rates of risk behavior peak in late adolescence rather than early or middle adolescence … Crime rises in teens until peaking at age 18, then drops steeply; substance use peaks at about age 20; automobile accidents and fatalities are highest in the late teens; sexually transmitted diseases (STDs) peak in the early twenties and two thirds of all STDs are contracted by people who are under 25 years old" (p. 321).

Sexual behavior escalates from early to late adolescence. At grade 9, approximately 28% of girls have had sexual intercourse compared to 38% of boys (Berk, 2010). By grade 12, approximately 62% of girls compared to 65% of boys have had sexual intercourse. Unfortunately, one in six teens who are sexually active will have an STD. Between 750,000 and 850,000 U.S. teens become pregnant each year, with 40% of these pregnancies ending in an abortion and 86% being to those who are unmarried (Berk, 2010). The United States has one of the highest pregnancy rates compared to other countries. Pregnancy rates among 15 to 19-year-old girls in the U.S. are over 75 per 1,000 females compared to 40 in Canada and 10 in Japan (Berk, 2010).

Adolescent substance abuse is another prominent problem. In 2012, alcohol was abused by 11% of 8th graders, 27.6% of 10th graders, and 41.5% of 12th graders. Illicit drugs were used by 7.7% of 8th graders, 18.6% of 10th graders, and 25.2% of 12th graders (National Institute on Drug Abuse (NIDA), 2012). Marijuana is the most frequently used illicit drug, with 6.5% of 12th graders using marijuana every day in 2012, compared to 5.1% in 2007. Drug abuse can have profound, unchangeable impacts on a critical period of the developing brain and body. Specifically, drugs reduce the number of dopamine receptors on the reward circuit and prevent substance abusers from experiencing pleasure. Consequently, adolescent drug abusers feel flat, lifeless, and depressed as well as lose cognitive ability. Unless treatment is provided, they will return to drugs to feel pleasure (NIDA, 2012).

In order to decrease risky behavior, adolescents need intrapersonal and interpersonal motivation, environmental controls, and self-control. According to Dahl and Hariri (2005), self-control is now conceptualized as involving cognitive inhibitory control (e.g. thought stopping), behavioral skills of emotion regulation (e.g. push button technique), and action monitoring (e.g. activity scheduling).

Social

The social hallmark of adolescence is peer interaction. As part of the individuation process, adolescents de-idealize their parents and shift their behavioral guidance from their parents to their peers. Although they have fewer "best friends," there is more intimacy, trust, and self-disclosure, and loyalty. Consequently, friends become more similar in identity status, aspirations, politics, and deviant behavior (Berk, 2010). Girls prefer to get together to "just talk" while boys prefer to get together for activities. Small groups of 5–7 good friends who are similar in interests and social status form cliques. Crowds are made up of several cliques with membership based on reputation and stereotype. Adolescents tend to begin dating within these crowds, moving from recreational group activities to more intimacy. Adolescents who date too early tend to engage in more risky behavior of drug use, sex, and delinquency, and achieve poor academic results (Berk, 2010).

Social development also entails moral development. Kohlberg (1981) created a six-stage model of moral development and believed that adolescents are between stage three and stage four. In stage three, moral reasoning is motivated by interpersonal cooperation so the adolescent can be seen as a "good boy" or "good girl". In stage four, moral reasoning is motivated by commitment to maintain social order by the ability to perceive abstract normative systems. Although adolescents' morality is still linked to laws and social norms, they have a more sophisticated understanding of why such laws and norms are important. Adolescents' moral reasoning is influenced by supportive parents, discussions of moral concerns, just educational environments, peer interactions, religious environments, and culture (Berk, 2010).

In summary, both biology and environment influence adolescents' physical, neurophysiological, cognitive, emotional, behavioral, and social development. "Genes bias how the brain processes information and thus color individuals' experiences and responses to their environment ... yet it is the interaction of the biological changes with the social influences that enable and promote behaviors" (Dahl & Hariri, 2005, pp. 376, 379). This finding implies that play therapists can create positive social influences for adolescents within AGT to steer them in a productive direction, no matter how narrow biology and previous environments made their passageway. Other developmental implications for goals, strategies, and activities will be discussed below.

Activity Group Therapy Origins and Rationale

Origins

AGT for children was a treatment started in 1943 by Slavson, a social worker with a Freudian psychoanalytic theoretical orientation. In his model, he carefully selected seven or eight adolescents for a group, allowed them free time with crafts or games, and ended sessions with a meal (Slavson, 1944). As an AGT group leader, Slavson was permissive rather than authoritarian and respected the individuality of each child. He believed this positive attitude along with emphasis of constructive achievement, development of skills, and consistency within sessions decreased children's anxiety related to their early intra-familial conflicts. Slavson helped dependent children by gradually withdrawing support so they would form child-to-child relationships and find security within self. The free environment facilitated children to release suppressed impulses so they could expand their inner life and strengthen their egos. Slavson found that rhythmic swings from hyperactivity to a state of equilibrium marked points of personal integration and emotional growth. "The 'instigators' in the group enable the more inhibited members to obtain catharsis during the periods of hyperactivity while the 'neutralizers' supply the group with social controls" (Vander, 1946, p. 552). Schiffer (1952) worked closely with Slavson and continued to promote "AGT as the treatment of choice with a majority of latency-age children" (Schiffer, 1977, p. 211). Consequently, AGT became a prominent model in public schools in the 1940s and 1950s.

In the 1960s, Ginott (1961), a classroom teacher and child psychotherapist, was another major promoter of AGT. However, unlike Slavson, he practiced from a CCPT approach. He saw AGT as a compromise between play therapy and traditional talk therapy for children aged 10–13 (Bratton & Ferebee, 1999). Ginott's primary contribution to the AGT movement was providing specific guidance for member selection (discussed later) and therapeutic limit-setting. He believed it was the therapist's responsibility to prevent children from experiencing ridicule in group therapy by stating "group members are not for ridiculing." Such limit-setting created freedom from fear so children would have emotional space to engage in growth-producing interactions.

Scheidlinger (1977) continued to promote AGT in the 1970s. He stated AGT prevented "the checker syndrome" in which therapists would play checkers every session with adolescents who refused traditional talk therapy. Scheidlinger believed the permissive environment of AGT allowed for the expression of feelings and fantasies through play and action in a manner that allowed for corrective emotional experiences with group members. In the 1980s and 1990s, numerous therapists described AGT case studies with various populations such as sexually abused adolescents (Celano, 1990), inpatient psychiatric patients (Lev, 1983), and girls with family losses (Roos & Jones, 1982).

Fortunately, in the new millennium, a surge of quantitative and qualitative research on the effectiveness of AGT occurred. For example, Troester's (2002) content analysis illustrated increased social interactions in a group of six adolescent boys from session one, in which there was minimal one-on-one subgroup interaction, through session 28, in which there was complex interaction of all members who formed a group as a whole. Packman and Bratton (2003) reported a statistically significant improvement in learning disabled preadolescents' behavior problems after AGT when compared to a control group. Paone, Packman, Maddux, and Rothman (2008) found a statistically significant difference in the moral reasoning of adolescents who received AGT compared to those who received traditional talk therapy. Gann (2010) described a qualitative analysis of hip-hop AGT with adolescents from a psychoanalytic perspective. Earls' (2011) research of Social Skills Group Play Therapy with adolescent African-American males revealed a statistically significant increase in positive self concept and decrease in anger and disruptive behavior for those in the treatment group compared to the control group. Hopefully, more researchers will examine the efficacy of AGT with adolescents in the coming years.

Rationale

As indicated above, the first rationale for AGT is that approximately 80 years of clinical practice and current research indicates that it is an effective approach for play therapists to use with adolescents (Gallo-Lopez & Schaefer, 2005).

A second rationale for AGT is that it meets adolescents' developmental needs. Their physical needs of discharging energy are met through stimulating gross motor activities. Therapeutic interaction can provide group members a sense of universality and acceptance of physical body changes (i.e., height and weight gain, puberty, acne, etc.). From a neurophysiological standpoint, AGT can reinforce neuro-pathways for affect regulation, particularly anxiety. "A key feature of anxiety is impaired learning of cues that signal safety versus threat and unlearning of cues that signal threat when the association no longer exists (i.e., extinction)" (Casey et al., 2010, p. 229). AGT facilitates face-to-face interactions in a fun environment for adolescents. The play therapist can help adolescents accurately interpret signals of safety and threat in real time; thereby relieving their anxiety. Play therapists also act as a synaptic bridge from adolescents' amygdale to their prefrontal cortex by facilitating reasoning, insight, and safe behavior with other group members.

Cognitive developmental needs of adolescents are met in AGT by asking participants to engage in and process activities that require abstract thinking such as problem-solving, perspective-taking, and reflective insight. Adolescents' behavioral developmental needs are met in AGT through the process of reality-testing. When adolescents become impulsive, offensive, or engage in risk-taking, peer and therapist feedback can motivate them to modify their behavior in exchange for social acceptance (Ginott, 1961). AGT also meets adolescents' social-emotional developmental needs for peer interactions in a positive environment. Participating in fun activities with peers can decrease depression (Wainscott, 2006). Troester (2002) summarized other socio-emotional benefits of AGT as follows:

> Adolescents transfer attachment from parents to friends, and those friendships are a crucial developmental factor in regard to working through identity concerns, building their sense of self-worth, developing skills for managing emotional adjustment, and determining long-term developmental outcomes, such as the quality of adult relationships and psychological well-being.

(p. 426)

A final rationale for AGT is that it promotes playfulness, a desirable personality trait of many adolescents. Playfulness projects spontaneous, carefree fun to friends and potential romantic partners, and thus is an adaptive survival mechanism. Play allows adolescents freedom to move back and forth along the developmental continuum from acting like a child to acting like an adult (Gallo-Lopez & Schaefer, 2005). This process helps adolescents to achieve needed individuation from adults so that they can be successful adults within their own pack of peers. In short, AGT provides a fun environment in which adolescents seeking stimulation can soar.

Preparation

Selection of Group Members

As indicated in earlier chapters, potential members for any type of group play therapy should have a pregroup screening interview. The primary requirement for group participation is a "social hunger" or a desire to participate and an ability to establish relationships (Slavson, 1948). According to Berg et al. (2006), adolescents with the following presenting problems would be appropriate for AGT:

• Difficulty with social and peer relationships.
• Impulse control and other behavioral problems.
• Poor self-esteem.
• Lack of motivation.
• Limited coping skills in adjusting to life.

In contrast, adolescents who would be excluded from AGT are those who have severe cognitive limitations, paranoia, extreme narcissism, psychosis, extreme aggression, sexually acting out, attachment disorders, or inability to tolerate rapidly changing environments (Slavson & Schiffer, 1975). Ginott (1961) recommended selecting group members with dissimilar presenting problems as their unbiased perspective allows them to have a corrective influence on each other. For example, one 13-year-old boy who was grieving the death of his grandfather said to another group member "If you get the flu, you could die." The other group member who sought therapy due to his parents' divorce responded with confidence "Well half my school friends and I had the flu but we didn't die. Don't be so worried." As illustrated, group members who are not struggling with the same problem communicate objectivity in a manner that filters through psychological defenses of other adolescents. Ginott also recommended selecting group members who do not have contact with each other outside of group therapy so that old roles, attitudes, and behaviors can be replaced with new ones more readily.

Group members should be similar in gender, chronological age and developmental age not more than 1 year apart. They should also be balanced based on personalities that complement each other in a therapeutic manner (Slavson, 1945). Adolescents who are instigators (i.e., provide catalyst and stimulate positive or negative activity) should be balanced with neutralizers (i.e., counteracts negative activity and calms interactions) and followers (i.e., floating or weak identities that succumb to stronger). Smith and Smith (1999) encouraged play therapists to conduct an individual session with each adolescent and then use their intuitive sense for placing adolescents in a group.

The Activity Room

The activity room should be "not too big" as this can lead to hyperactivity, "not too small" as this can contribute to anger and aggression, but rather "just right" with approximately 300 square feet for five children. This amount of space allows for roaming, exploring, and creativity for all members. Since few play therapists have such a large space, a well-planned room of 200 square feet would suffice for three or four adolescents.

Materials for AGT need to be carefully selected to allow for creative expression. Standard items for AGT include a puppet theater, woodworking table, sandtray and miniatures, a multipurpose game table (i.e., pool, air hockey, ping pong), shelves to store age-appropriate games and toys, crafts, easel, paints, dress-up items, musical instruments, sports equipment, and tables large enough for more than one child to work on a project at a time (Bratton & Ferebee, 1999; Ginott, 1975; Slavson, 1945). For a more extensive list, see Table 11.1. Smith and Smith (1999) recommend materials be organized on shelves and bins according to categories as follows:

- Expressive arts and crafts (i.e., colored paper, markers, clay, pipe cleaners).
- Symbolic acting out (i.e., puppets, dress-up clothing, dolls, sandtray miniatures).
- Skill-building materials and equipment (i.e., Lego, do-it-yourself building project kits, model airplane, beads, jewelry materials).
- Gross motor games (i.e., basketball, bowling sets, plastic dart set, foam bats).
- Commercial and therapeutic board games (i.e., checkers, break-the-ice, talking, doing, and feeling game, the ungame).

Table 11.1   Categories and Lists of Materials for AGT (Smith & Smith, 1999, pp. 262–264)

Construction Supplies:	*Sports Equipment:*
Workbench with vise	Basketball goal for door
Basic tools: saw, hammer, screwdriver	Various balls: Nerf, volleyball, basketball, Nerf football
Building supplies: lumber, nails, screws, bolts	
Glue gun	Training gloves (like boxing gloves)
Wood glue and tapes: masking, duct, scotch	Large vinyl bop bag (sand in bottom)
Nonelectric hand drill	Balls and catcher's mitts coated with Velcro hook-and-loop fastening
Woodburning set and simple wood-carving tools	
	Home type trampoline
	Badminton rackets and birdies
Art Supplies:	Whiffle ball and scoops
Paints: tempera, watercolors, special acrylics (for special projects)	*Games:*
Large to small paint brushes, sponge brushes, and sponge pieces	Checkers, chess
	Deck of cards
Oil pastels, colored chalk, and colored pencils	Labyrinth
Markers of various sizes	Pick-up sticks
Various paper suitable for various media	Skittles (spinning top with string)
Colored tissue	Small table-top pinball game (battery run)
Posterboard	Foos ball, Ping-Pong, or 2′ × 4′ pool table
Glues: glue gun, Modge Podge, spray shellac, spray adhesive, fabric glue, rubber cement, white glue	*Additional Furnishings:*
Various tapes	Floor pillows
Various magazines	Shelf for safekeeping of unfurnished projects
Potter's clay and colored clay suitable for drying or for baking in regular oven	Dual work and snack table
	Throw rug (for gathering)
Colored beads, feathers, glitter, scraps of felt, yarn, and fabric	Old quilt or blanket
Plaster of Paris gauze strips for facial masks	

(continued)

Table 11.1   Continued

Music-Making Instruments:	Dramatic Play:
Old guitar (garage sale type)	Hats
Tambourine	Makeup
Various drums	Jewelry
Battery-powered keyboard	Scarves, wigs, ties, vests
Sandtrays and Sandtray Miniatures:	Masks
	Props-feathers, wand, baton
Dry sandtray	*Unique Crafts:*
Wet sandtray	
Sandtray miniatures	Group journal books
Micro machines and micro soldiers	Jewelry making
Cooking Supplies and Ingredients:	Leather making
	Copper work
Electric skillet	Mosaic work
Egg beater or hand-held electric mixer	Embroidery thread for sewing, bracelets, and
Paper plates	necklaces
Mixing utensils and bowls	T-shirt painting
Flour, sugar, salt, food coloring, tubes of icing,	Tie dye
decorative sugars	Mask-making
Toaster oven with temperature range (garage	Papier-mâché
sale item)	Clay sculpting
Vinyl tablecloth	Bread dough objects
Brownie, cookie, and pancake mixes	
Small aluminum baking pans	

If possible, setting up these materials in a separate room for AGT is more desirable than just adding items to a typical play therapy room used for young children. Adolescents who are desperately attempting to establish themselves as adults can be offended and thus resistant if they are asked to participate in a "little kids'" room on a regular basis. On the other hand, Riviere (2005) stated that a typical office with a desk and computer can be intimidating to adolescents. Instead, adolescents prefer a separate room with the materials described above and a couch and loveseat.

Group Format

There are three main approaches to group format. Unstructured groups, as recommended by Slavson (1944), allow adolescents to have free play with toys and crafts during the entire session. In an unstructured approach, adolescents choose activities on their own accord and interact with others in their own time. In contrast, structured groups, as recommended by Schaefer and Reid (1986), are planned and directed. In a structured approach, the play therapist directs adolescents in what to do and when to do it. An integrative approach of both unstructured and structured was recommended by Gil (1994) and Smith and Smith (1999).

In an integrative approach, play therapists divide the session into (a) directed group activity, (b) free play time, and (c) snack and talk time (Smith & Smith, 1999). Structured time reduces group members' anxiety, encourages interaction early on, and provides stimulation. Unstructured time allows adolescents to explore, experiment, and make decisions with other members (Smith & Smith, 1999). Snack and talk time allows the play therapist to facilitate group discussions, awareness of group dynamics, insight into self and others, development of pro-social skills, and affirmation of positive changes. The snack and talk time gives adolescents an opportunity to share their voice, thereby activating their internal power to shape positive social interactions. Adolescents are encouraged to participate in making their snack and cleaning it up. They may even take turns hosting the snack. Before enjoying the snack, group members sit together in a circle on the floor or at a table. This circle creates a family atmosphere so adolescents are more likely to share thoughts and feelings. The snack time also provides a closing ritual.

The balance of time between structured activities, unstructured activities, and snack fluctuates over the course of treatment. In the forming stage of treatment, group members are usually more comfortable when there is more time on structured activities. As treatment progresses into the working stage, they may have developed enough cohesion and openness to prefer more time in unstructured and snack time.

Regardless of the group format selected, play therapists are to address problems when they arise. Play therapists should reflect feelings, encourage members to solve their own problems, suggest problem-solving strategies only when needed, and affirm pro-social resolution. Therapeutic limit-setting of reflecting the feeling, communicating the limit, and targeting an alternative is reserved for when there is potential harm to people, property, or group process.

Self-Preparation

Play therapists may have experienced storm and stress during their own adolescence. In order to mitigate counter-transference, self-exploration and healing through therapeutic activities described below is recommended. It is helpful for play therapists to reflect on who they were as adolescents compared to present time and who was their nemesis compared to present time. Recognizing gradual growth in self and adolescent friends can motivate play therapists to be patient with adolescents.

Clothing and hair style can send an immediate signal to adolescents as to whether the play therapist is relaxed, relatable, and trustworthy. Adolescents may perceive play therapists who wear formal business attire (i.e., suits, ties, business skirts, and other clothing that must be dry cleaned) as "one of them" (i.e., too formal or uptight) (Riviere, 2005). However, if play therapists wear comfortable professional clothing (termed "business casual") from a store that market to adolescents and obtain an updated hair style, then adolescents' first impression may be "this person understands me." Being familiar with pop culture (i.e., celebrities, music, expressions, etc.) will also enable play therapists to relate with adolescents.

Self-disclosure is a therapeutic skill that should be used judiciously for the benefit of clients. Adolescents may be much less guarded if play therapists participate in AGT activities with them. Play therapists' participation helps overcome adolescents' bravado of "I'm too cool" to engage in creative activities (Riviere, 2005). When play therapists participate in activities, they model appropriate risk-taking and encourage emotional reciprocity. Of course, play therapists should not work out their own emotional issues during the process but rather participate at a level where they are able to respond therapeutically to adolescents.

In order to maintain emotional contact with adolescents, play therapists must be consistently warm, trustworthy, and predictable (Riviere, 2005). Adolescents may have experienced multiple episodes of rejection and betrayal from friends, dating partners, and family members. As a result, they may use distance, anger, sarcasm, lack of cooperation, and insults as defense mechanisms from being hurt again. Rather than being offended by such behavior (i.e., "taking it personally"), play therapists must consistently convey the three core conditions of unconditional positive regard, empathy, and genuineness with adolescents (Rogers, 1951).

Common pitfalls of engaging in sarcasm, teasing, or over-exerting control can fracture trust. Play therapists can maintain trust by modeling a therapeutic response such as reflecting feelings, facilitating understanding of intent, setting therapeutic limits, building self-esteem, and using light-hearted humor appropriately.

ESTEPHANIE: Gee, Miss, what happened to your hair? Did you go through a blizzard?

PLAY THERAPIST: Estephanie, you don't like my hair today and are trying to give me a suggestion, like perhaps I should go see Rodolfo Valentin [a famous New York hair stylist].

ESTEPHANIE: Yeah, and while you're at it, get some new shoes.

PLAY THERAPIST: You know a lot about fashion. You enjoy looking "fly." Perhaps we could work that into a creative activity next week.

ESTEPHANIE: Well, maybe we should tell Maria how to dress 'cause she dresses like a trashy whore.

MARIA: F*** you, slut.

PLAY THERAPIST: Maria, you are angry at Estephanie. Estephanie, you don't like Maria's clothes. But in our activity room, people are not for insulting with words or actions. You can choose to use different words to communicate a constructive message.

ESTEPHANIE: Well, I was just trying to give Maria some free fashion advice.

MARIA: Well, I don't want it from you.

PLAY THERAPIST: Estephanie, you wanted to help out Maria. Maria, you aren't ready to hear it just yet. Sometimes people need time to have positive experiences together before they can trust each other enough to hear advice. Maybe then we can all take a trip to see Rodolfo Valentin!

In the interaction above, the play therapist did not take the insult personally but rather responded to the adolescent's intent with light-hearted humor. Any deeper analysis or limit-setting at this point may have created a barrier between adolescent and play therapist. When the first adolescent insulted another group member, then the play therapist set a therapeutic limit by reflecting the feelings, communicating a limit, and targeting an alternative. In the final response, the play therapist facilitated understanding by identifying the dynamics of trust and the general context in which it is most helpful. These therapeutic skills can be implemented during expressive and creative art activities as needed.

Expressive and Creative Art Activities

Expressive and creative art activities for adolescents include drawing, painting, sculpting, music, dance movement, drama, writing, phototherapy, collages, sandplay, imagery, fantasy, improvisation, puppetry, and woodworking (Gallo-Lopez & Schaefer, 2005; Smith & Smith, 1999). "Through these various expressive art forms the individual has the opportunity to take elements of his or her own personality and restructure them into new forms" (Smith & Smith, 1999, p. 200). Play therapists are advised to begin with less threatening, contained, and controlled activities such as collages and gradually progress to more open expressive activities such as drama therapy. Numerous expressive art, puppet play, and sandtray activities are described in Chapters 8, 9, and 10, respectively. Do-it-yourself projects, woodworking, beads for necklaces, and other arts and crafts are self-explanatory. Thus, the following section will focus on additional activities that adolescents enjoy within group stages of forming, working, and closure.

Forming Stage

During the forming stage, adolescent group members tend to hesitate before interacting in an attempt to evaluate other members' personalities, behaviors, and power for the purpose of determining where they fit in the social matrix. Many adolescents will experience anxiety, masked in different forms as distance, resistance, or over-dependence. The role of the play therapist is to alleviate anxiety by promoting safety, establishing a group identity, clarifying roles, and developing norms (Van Velsor, 2004). In order to facilitate this process, the play therapists can lead group members in discussion of the rules and active ice breakers before introducing structured activities.

The Rules

Since confidentiality is needed to maintain a safe environment for AGT, it is helpful to begin the group sessions with "the rules" activity (Riviere, 2005). Each group member is given five 3″ × 5″ index cards. The play therapist says "together we will create rules for our time together so that we can create a safe and respectful environment. The rules must be realistic, doable, and stated in the positive such as "do take turns talking" rather than "don't interrupt." The play therapist instructs group members to write down one rule on each card and to either draw a symbol or find a magazine picture that represents the rule on the back of the index card. For example, for a rule such as "be supportive of others' feelings," a group member could draw a sad face with a check mark by it. The play therapist participates in the activity and writes essential rules such as keeping conversations confidential, keeping bodies safe, telling the truth, and saying things in an encouraging way. Each group member lays out their cards with the symbol facing up. Other group members try to guess what the rule is. Then the group as a whole consolidates rules and decides which ones to keep. The rules are written on clean paper for each member to sign, indicating that they will follow the rules.

Active Ice Breaker

The purpose of an active ice breaker is to decrease group members' anxiety, increase rapport, release energy, and provide focus for group members. Beginning each session with an active ice breaker provides a predictable routine. Numerous active ice breakers have been described elsewhere (Johnson, 2012; Ragsdale & Saylor, 2007). One active ice breaker called "Circle Common Run" was developed by this author (Baggerly) to identify commonalities among members. The play therapist prepares a list of yes or no questions regarding individual and family characteristics (i.e., age is 13; have brothers; live with your father, etc.), interests (i.e., plays soccer; listens to hip-hop; goes to church, etc.), experiences (i.e., traveled out of state; fought at school; teased by a bully), and feelings (i.e., loves pet dog; angry at father; sad that someone close died; hurt by ex-love). Group members stand in a circle. When the play therapist reads an item that applies to a member, group members run or walk around a circle in various ways (run with hands on head, run backwards, walk slowly, hop on left foot, etc.). For example, the play therapist may say "if you play basketball, run around the circle like you are dribbling a basketball" or "if you are angry at your brother or sister, walk around the circle punching the sky." This active ice breaker can help adolescents release physical energy and gain a sense of universality.

The Theraplay® Institute (2005) has described numerous activities for facilitating groups of children that can be used as ice breakers. One activity is the "name game," in which participants sit in a circle and the first person says "my name is __," using any tone of voice or intonation. The other group members say "your name is __," imitating the tone and intonation three times (The Theraplay® Institute, 2005, p. 66). In another activity, called "row, row, row your boat," participants form two lines and sit across from each other so that pairs are facing together (The Theraplay® Institute, 2005, p. 7). Partners clasp hands and row back and forth as they sing "row, row, row your boat" at varying speeds of fast and slow.

Who Am I? Collage

The purpose of the Who Am I? collage is for adolescents to reflect on, explore, and disclose their self-perception (Rubin, 2010). This activity can also identify commonalities among other members. The play therapist provides each member a poster board and an assortment of magazines (e.g., sports, entertainment, fashion, travel, news, etc.). Play therapists can ask businesses (i.e., doctors' offices, hair salons, etc.) to donate their magazines for this activity. Each member finds magazine pictures or online computer pictures that can be printed out to answer: (a) Who am I?; (b) What is my life purpose?; and (c) Where do I belong? Group members cut out pictures and paste them on the poster board. After 15–20 minutes, the play therapist asks each member to show which pictures they used to answer the questions. Then the play therapist asks other members to identify what they have in common. The play therapist may also identify moods such as happiness or loneliness that were reflected in the projects.

Working Stage

During the working stage, group members become comfortable enough to challenge each other, take on more responsibility, and cooperate with each other (Van Velsor, 2004). The role of the play therapist is to become a guide rather than the focal point so that group members' interactions with each other deepen. Since a supportive atmosphere has been consistently experienced, adolescents are more likely to openly share. In so doing, they continue to explore their "me identity" and their new found "we identity." The following activities can facilitate metaphoric thinking and abreaction during the working stage.

Music Therapy

Music is a meaningful medium that can unite adolescents. Hadley and Yancy (2012) identified several ways that music, particularly rap and hip-hop, can be used in therapy with adolescents. These methods include listening and discussing, performing, creating, and improvising.

"Rap music can function as a cathartic release of emotions that have been calcified after years of refusing to face them. The function of rap music as a surrogate voice speaks to the reality of the social interconnectedness of voices and how particular lyrical content and forms of voicing/rapping speak to shared pain, angst, and joy" (Hadley & Yancy, 2012, p. xxxiv).

Play therapists can ask adolescents to share a song that represents their life experiences, attitudes, relationships, self-perception, society's perception of them, their perception of society, and their future (Hadley & Yancy, 2012). After listening to a member's song, play therapists ask group members to discuss lyrics that were meaningful to them. The group also discusses how these lyrics reflect aspects of self, society, and their future.

For example, in one AGT, a 16-year-old girl shared a song by Kelly Clarkson called "Stronger" and focused on lyrics of "What doesn't kill you makes you stronger. Doesn't mean I'm lonely when I'm alone." She related these lyrics to her experience of not being selected for the cheerleading team. Another group member related it to his parent's divorce. The play therapist identified the human universal experience of loss leading to strength for the future. After sharing her specific song, the play therapist asked group members to perform actions to the song lyrics that represented their individual experiences of loss leading to strength. The actions were video recorded with a computer so members could see themselves in their own music video.

Drama Therapy

According to Oaklander (1988), "drama is a natural means of helping children find and give expression to lost and hidden parts of themselves, and to build strength and self-hood" (p. 139). Drama allows adolescents to play out their wishes, fears, fantasies, and realities (Gallo-Lopez, 2005). Originating from Jacob Moreno's psychodrama, drama therapy uses theater techniques to foster personal growth and improve mental health. Drama therapy emphasizes the process rather than a product of a formal play. As adolescents play out the roles they have, do not have, and wish to have, they formulate their identity (Gallo-Lopez, 2005). To implement drama therapy, a variety of props are needed, including hats, ties, scarves, jewelry, badges, sunglasses, telephones, masks, capes, boas, etc.

Drama therapy begins with a warm-up activity such as "pass the hat," in which each member selects a different hat, acts out a character (i.e., cowboy, old lady, etc.), and passes the hat to another member to act out the character (Gallo-Lopez, 2005). An alternative warm-up activity is "my superhero," in which each member acts out their personal hero before, during, and after a challenge they faced. For example, if an adolescent's hero is Spiderman, he may act as a curious boy who then uses his powers to fight an evil scientist in an effort to win the girl he loves.

After the warm up, adolescents participate in "the action" or main activity. Gallo-Lopez (2005) recommends inspiring enactment and role playing through story starters such as "The Family Secret," "The Family Crisis," or "The Great Escape" (p. 87). Another action activity is "Adolescent turmoil and triumph," in which group members select props and other group members to act out a personal experience of turmoil or a personal experience of triumph. For example, a 16-year-old male acted out his experience at his father's funeral. He directed a friend to lie down in a mock casket while he played an exaggerated preacher who commanded his father to rise back to life.

Closure in drama therapy prepares members to return to the real world through calming, reflection, and feedback (Gallo-Lopez, 2005). The purpose is to de-role adolescents from their character by talking about the character in the third person, writing a letter to the character, or identifying the differences between self and the character (Gallo-Lopez, 2005). In the above example, the teenager voiced his yearning for power to make his father come back to life like the preacher. However, he did not want to be seen to be as obnoxious as the role he had played. Group members affirmed his right to be sad and his desire to be powerful. Then the group discussed strategies for him to feel connected to his father, such as attending religious ceremonies, talking to him as if he was on the phone, and lifting weights, an activity they had done together.

Closure of Treatment

Closure activities toward the end of AGT treatment are essential to authenticate the value of relationships formed in treatment and to prepare adolescents to generalize their new working models of self and others. Ideally, play therapists will inform adolescents of the upcoming ending of AGT four sessions before it ends. This will give time for play therapists to role-model healthy grieving and celebrate therapeutic progress (Riviere, 2005).

Poetry

Poetry or inspirational messages can allow for a deeper and more honest type of communication with adolescents (Taylor & Abell, 2005). The sublimatory nature of poetry allows for creative expression of feelings, fears, and desires. To promote a therapeutic and hopeful ending, play therapists ask adolescents to find or create a positive poem or an inspirational story to give as a gift to other members in the next to last meeting. The play therapist models by sharing a poem or inspirational story of hope such as a caterpillar struggling to become a butterfly.

Give a Hand

Transitional objects are a powerful way for group members to remember each other and acknowledge their progress together (Riviere, 2005; Tabin, 2005). One transitional activity is called "Give a Hand." Each group member writes their name at the top of a piece of paper and traces their hand print below. The group members pass their paper around the circle so that each person can write a few words of appreciation in the hand. After each member receives their own paper, group members take turns verbally expressing their appreciation.

Conclusion

Although Hall identified adolescence as a period of "storm and stress," it can also be a period in which adolescents are seeking stimulation to soar. Play therapists need to understand adolescents' unique development, including (a) the physical hallmark of puberty; (b) the neuro-physiological hallmark of amygdale dominance; (c) the cognitive hallmark of abstract thought; (d) the emotional hallmark of moodiness; (e) the behavioral mark of risky behavior; and (f) the social hallmark of peer interaction. This understanding will increase play therapists' empathy and direct them in creating activities that meet adolescents' developmental needs.

AGT has a long history of being identified as effective in treating adolescents, beginning with Slavson (1943) and continuing with Ginott (1961), Scheidlinger (1977), and contemporary play therapy researchers. Not only does AGT meet adolescents' developmental needs, it is also a fun and appealing modality that promotes playfulness, a desirable personality trait of many adolescents.

Play therapists prepare for AGT by selecting compatible group members via pre-group screening interviews. An activity room of approximately 200–300 square feet is prepared with creative expressive materials organized by category. Play therapists select one of three group formats, either an unstructured group, structured group, or integrative group. No matter which format is selected, basic play therapy skills of reflecting feelings, encouraging problem-solving, and setting therapeutic limits are implemented. Play therapists also prepare themselves through self-reflection of their own adolescence and being up to date in clothing, hair style, and pop culture. They must be consistently warm, trustworthy, and predictable even when adolescents insult them.

Activities for the forming stage of AGT include creating the rules, active ice breakers, and "Who Am I? Collage". Activities for the working stage include music therapy and drama therapy. Finally, closure activities include poetry and "Give a Hand" transitional object. By implementing AGT, play therapists will help adolescents seeking stimulation to soar.

12   Disaster Response Group Play Therapy Procedures

Children are one of the most vulnerable populations during and after disasters because they lack experience, skills, and resources to meet their physical and mental health needs (La Greca, Silverman, Vernberg, & Roberts, 2002). In 2010, the United States National Commission on Children and Disasters (NCCD) recommended to the President and Congress that "federal agencies and non-Federal partners should enhance predisaster preparedness and just-in-time training in pediatric disaster mental and behavioral health, including psychological first aid, bereavement support, and brief supportive interventions, for mental health professionals" (NCCD, 2010, p. 9). Play therapists are an important part of this national disaster preparedness and response effort because play therapy experience and skills can enhance standard disaster response approaches (Baggerly, 2006b). The purpose of this chapter is to prepare play therapists for disaster response by (a) identifying disaster descriptions and prevalence; (b) describing the impact of disasters on children; (c) discussing disaster response principles; and (d) explaining play-based disaster response interventions strategies for groups of children.

Disaster Descriptions and Prevalence

Disasters are defined as events that meet the following seven criteria: (a) destruction of property, injury, or loss of life; (b) identifiable beginning and end; (c) sudden and time-limited; (d) adversely affects a large group of people; (e) public event that impacts more than one family; (f) out of realm of ordinary experience; and (g) psychologically traumatic enough to induce stress in almost anyone (Rosenfeld, Caye, Ayalon, & Lahad, 2005). Natural disasters are categorized into five subgroups: geophysical (e.g., earthquakes, landslides); meteorological (e.g., tornados and hurricanes); hydrological (e.g., floods, tidal waves); climatological (e.g., drought, wildfire); and biological (e.g., epidemic) (Guha-Sapir, Vos, Below, & Ponserre, 2012). According to the World Health Organization Centre for Research on the Epidemiology of Disasters in 2011, a total of 332 natural disasters killed 30,773 people, affected 244.7 million others, and caused US$366.1 billion in economic damage (Guha-Sapir et al., 2012).

In contrast, so-called "man-made" disasters originate from human intent (e.g., war, terrorism, mass shootings) or human error (oil spills, nuclear leaks, plane crashes). UNICEF (2007) estimated that 1 billion children live in countries or territories affected by armed conflict; 300 million of these children were under 5 years old. An estimated 20 million children worldwide have fled their homes due to armed conflicts and human rights violations (UNICEF, 2007). Recent massive shootings in the U.S. (e.g., Sandy Hook Elementary School in Connecticut, Aurora movie theater in Colorado) have activated fear in untold numbers of children across the nation.

Due to this prevalence of natural and man-made disasters, millions of U.S. children may experience disaster-related symptoms. In fact, Becker-Blease, Turner, and Finkelhor (2010) conducted a representative sample survey of 2,030 U.S. children aged 2 to 17. They found that approximately 14% of respondents reported a lifetime exposure to a disaster and 4.1% in the past year. This estimate indicates that, of the nation's 74 million children, over 3 million will have been exposed to a disaster within the past year.

Impact of Disasters on Children

Both natural and man-made disasters can cause typical short-term and atypical long-term symptoms in children. It is important to distinguish between typical and atypical responses to determine which interventions are needed.

Typical Symptoms

After a disaster, children may experience short-term responses in five areas (Baggerly, 2010; Speier, 2000). In the cognitive realm, disasters can change children's beliefs and judgments, such as believing all rain storms will destroy their home (La Greca et al., 2002; Speier, 2000). Children may have difficulty concentrating or making decisions, which can impact academic performance. Baggerly and Ferretti (2008) found that hurricanes did not impact standardized test scores of students after the 2004 hurricanes in Florida. However, Pane, McCaffrey, Kalra, and Zhou (2008) found that students displaced in Louisiana after the 2005 hurricanes did have negative changes in their standardized test scores.

In the second realm of emotions and affect, disasters may hinder children's ability to manage their feelings of fear and anger, connect with others, feel worthy of life, and maintain a healthy self-esteem (La Greca et al., 2002; Speier, 2000). Young children may experience separation anxiety or exhibit fear of trauma reminders such as rain. For example, after a hurricane, a boy refused to take a bath for over a month because the family was hunkered down in the bathtub when the hurricane destroyed the roof of their house.

In the third realm of behavior, children impacted by disasters may experience social withdrawal, clinginess, hypervigilance, bed-wetting, belligerence, aggressiveness, or school refusal (Brymer et al., 2006; La Greca, 2008). Children may also engage in traumatic play reenactments (Terr, 1990). For example, boys in a hurricane shelter played hurricane by spinning around and knocking things over.

In the fourth realm of physical symptoms, children may have headaches, stomach aches, sleeplessness, or fatigue (Brymer et al., 2006; La Greca, 2008). The final realm is spirituality or worldview. Children may doubt their beliefs about God, their identity as a "carefree child," and their worldview (i.e., the world is a dangerous place). For example, one girl in a homeless shelter used a dart gun to shoot at a cross, saying "I'm zapping God like he zapped my family."

These typical symptoms tend to vary in prominence based on the age of the child (see Table 12.1). Again, most of these typical symptoms will resolve within a short time.

Speier (2000) stated, "Generally, most children recover from the frightening experiences associated with a disaster without professional intervention. Most simply need time to experience their world as a secure place again and their parents as nurturing caregivers who are also again in charge" (p. 9).

Table 12.1 Children's Trauma Responses by Age and Intervention Guidelines

Age	Typical trauma responses	Intervention guidelines
Preschool–2nd grade	Believes death is reversible Magical thinking Intense but brief grief responses Worries others will die Separation anxiety and excessive clinging Sleep terrors or nightmares Avoidance Regressive symptoms (e.g., thumb sucking, bed-wetting) Fear of the dark Reenactment through traumatic play	Give simple, concrete explanations as needed Provide physical closeness Allow expression through play Read story books: *A Terrible Thing Happened* *Brave Bart* *Don't Pop Your Cork on Monday*
3rd–6th grade	Asks lots of questions Begins to understand death is permanent Worries about own death Irrational fears Increased fighting and aggression Hyperactivity and inattentiveness Withdrawal from friends Depression Reenactment through traumatic play School refusal	Give clear, accurate explanations Allow expression through art, journaling Ready story books
Middle school	Physical symptoms of headache, stomach aches Wide range of emotions More verbal but still needs physical outlet Arguments, fighting Moodiness Depression	Be accepting of moodiness Be supportive and discuss when they are ready Groups with structured art activities or games
High school	Understands death is irreversible but believes won't happen to them Depression Risk-taking behaviors Alcohol and other drug use Lack of concentration Decline in responsible behavior Avoidance of developmentally appropriate separation (e.g., going to camp or college) Apathy Rebellion at home or school	Listen Encourage expression of feelings Groups with guiding questions and projects

Atypical Symptoms

Although these reactions to disasters typically resolve within 30 days, some children may experience severe and ongoing symptoms such as depression, anxiety, and Post Traumatic Stress Disorder (PTSD) for months and years if left untreated (Kronenberg et al., 2010). For example, moderate to very severe symptoms were reported by 55% of school-aged children 3 months after Hurricane Andrew and by 34% at 10 months post-disaster (La Greca, Silverman, Vernberg, & Prinstein, 1996). Similarly, 1 year after Hurricane Katrina, 61% of elementary school children living in high-impact areas screened positive for elevated PTSD symptoms (Jaycox et al., 2010). Approximately 2 years after Hurricane Katrina, 31% of parents surveyed reported their children had clinically diagnosed depression, anxiety, or behavior disorders and 18% reported notable decreases in academic achievement (Abramson, Stehling-Ariza, Garfield, & Redlener, 2008).

These atypical, severe symptoms occur due to the impact of a disaster on children's neurophysiology (La Greca, 2008; Perry, 2006). When a disaster threatens children's actual or perceived physical or psychological safety, their brains activate either an arousal response of "fight or flight" or a dissociative response of "freeze and surrender" (Perry, Pollard, Blakely, Baker, & Vigilante, 1995; van der Kolk, 2006). During this time, brain functioning decreases in Broca's area, which controls ability to speak, and in Wernicke's area, which controls ability to comprehend language (van der Kolk, 2006). Children, like adults, can become "scared speechless." Children may not be able to formulate the words for a narrative of the disaster-related traumatic event but they will encode an indelible picture of the event in their implicit memory. Some children enter an altered state during a traumatic event to manage the terror. During the altered state, children become fixated on one image such as their favorite toy being swept away or destroyed in the disaster. This terrifying mental picture may become a "fixed idea" in children's memory like a DVD stuck on pause (Baggerly, 2010). Children need to process and integrate their images of a traumatic event into their explicit memory. Otherwise, they may reexperience the trauma through intrusive images, attempt to avoid these frightening images and trauma-related stimuli; and/or exhibit increased arousal such as hypervigilance, posttraumatic play, or outbursts of anger (Gil, 2011; van der Kolk; 2006).

Screening for Typical vs. Atypical Symptoms

To discern which children are most likely to have atypical long-term symptoms after disasters, play therapists can seek answers to the following questions (Rosenfeld et al., 2005).

What were the characteristics of the disaster? Longer duration and higher intensity results in more severe symptoms (La Greca, 2008). Man-made disasters tend to result in more serious mental health problems because people's trust in social order has been violated (U.S. Department of Health and Human Services, 2004).

What was the child's exposure to the disaster? Closer exposure, and particularly perceived life threat, results in more severe symptoms (La Greca et al., 2010).

What are the characteristics of the student, including age, gender, and prior victimization? Females and younger children tend to have more severe symptoms, as do children with prior abuse or victimization (Becker-Blease et al., 2010).

What is the student's interpersonal, cultural, and social context? Children tend to mimic their parents and significant adults' reactions to a disaster. Parents who display excessive anxiety tend to have children who do so as well. Children with stronger interpersonal support from caring family members and peer support tend to have less severe symptoms (La Greca et al., 2010). Children from groups with less economic and socio-political power such as ethnic minorities and other marginalized populations tend to have more severe symptoms. Differing cultures and religions attribute different meaning and respond differently to a disaster. For example, some Mexican American Catholics may view a disaster as a consequence for a sin, while some European American Protestants may view the disaster as a random act of God.

What is the wider, social, political, and economic context, including disaster planning and relief efforts? Children who perceive and receive more support and resources from community members, government agencies, nongovernment organizations, tend to have less severe symptoms. In contrast, children who perceive the government is against them may have more severe symptoms (Abramson et al., 2008).

In addition to using these questions to identify children at-risk, play therapists can screen children by using assessments such as the *Child's Reaction to Traumatic Events Scale-Revised* (Jones, Fletcher, & Ribbe, 2002) or the *Disaster Experiences Questionnaire* (Scheeringa, 2005). PTSD symptoms can be measured by the *Trauma Symptom Checklist for Young Children* (Briere, 1996). Other recommendations for assessment instruments are available from the National Children Traumatic Stress Network at www.nctsnet.org

Disaster Intervention Principles

Given these distressing symptoms that children may experience after a disaster, play therapists may be tempted to rush to provide interventions to alleviate children's suffering. However, play therapists must be resolute in holding to emergency mental health guiding principles during early stages of a crisis and later recovery. A synthesis of these principles from the National Child Traumatic Stress Network (Brymer et al., 2006), Speier (2000), World Health Organization (2003), Baggerly (2006b; 2010) are provided below.

- Only deploy to a disaster relief area when invited by an established government agency (e.g., Federal Emergency Management Agency or school district) or a nongovernment organization (e.g., American Red Cross, local church).
- Comply with the Incident Command Structure by registering with those in charge and following their guidelines.
- Collaborate with other professionals to schedule and implement children's interventions.
- Maintain a calm, non-anxious presence by managing internal anxiety through deep breathing, positive self-talk, and proactive self-care.
- Convey the expectation that most children will have a normal recovery so as not to over pathologize children's understandable and expected responses (Brymer et al., 2006).
- Maintain flexibility in your intervention protocol, allowing for variations to accommodate different environments, cultures, and personal characteristics.

- Respond in a way that is consistent with the child's level of development.
- Be aware of how the child's emotional status differs from their typical mood. Is the child actively afraid or withdrawn when they are usually outgoing and friendly?
- Determine if the child is comfortable/secure about his/her current surroundings and those of his or her parents, and other significant persons/pets.
- Convey the view that children are capable of positive self-direction if given unconditional positive regard, genuineness, and empathy (Landreth, 2012).

Play therapists who follow these principles will be regarded as a valuable team member by other disaster responders and a trustworthy helper by children and family members.

Play-Based Group Interventions

After a disaster, play therapists may be involved in the immediate post-impact phase (i.e., immediately after an event to a few weeks), short-term recovery phase (i.e., a few weeks to first year after an event), and/or long-term recovery phase (i.e., first year or more after an event). Interventions are selected based on the phase of disaster (La Greca & Silverman, 2009). In the immediate post-impact phase, all children receive Psychological First Aid and large group interventions to reduce typical symptoms. In the short-term recovery phase, children with ongoing typical symptoms and severe atypical symptoms receive small group play-based interventions. In the return to life phase, children with persistent atypical symptoms receive small group play therapy.

Immediate Post-Impact Phase

During the immediate post-impact phase, disaster survivors congregate at shelters or facilities for physical safety and to acquire practical assistance. The focus is on immediate needs and safety. Psychological interventions are brief and present-focused with the goal of reducing symptoms and long-term difficulties (La Greca & Silverman, 2009). In this phase, Psychological First Aid (PFA) is considered the treatment of choice (La Greca & Silverman, 2009). "PFA is an evidence-informed modular approach to help children, adolescents, adults, and families ... designed to reduce the initial distress caused by traumatic events and to foster short- and long-term adaptive functioning and coping" (Brymer et al., 2006, p. 5). This intervention is delivered one-on-one in about 15–20 minutes, usually at a disaster relief center, medical facility, or near the site of the disaster after safety has been established. Baggerly and Mescia (2005) developed a modified PFA approach for children in the C^3ARE model.

C^3ARE. This acronym stands for Check, Connect, Comfort, Access, Refer, and Educate.

Check—responders check the scene to make sure it is safe; check in with the formal structure and people in charge; check self to ensure calmness; check to see which child may need interventions the most.

Connect—connect with the child survivor and their parent or guardian through statements such as "Hi my name is Jennifer. This is my puppet Shep, the Sheepdog. I'm here with the team helping out today. Is it O.K. if I visit with you a few minutes? Would you like to pet Shep? What's your name? Who is here with you today?"

Comfort—calm and stabilize the child by asking "What can I do to help you feel more comfortable? Would you like some water or a snack? What do you usually do to calm yourself? I know some ways to help kids calm down. Would you like to learn?" Teach stabilization techniques such as "deep" breathing and progressive muscle relaxation.

Assess—observational assessments are done to monitor child survivor's physical and behavioral health status and to determine coping and functioning. Helpful questions are "Is anything in your body hurting or feeling strange right now? Can you show me your drawings or tell me a story about what happened?" Children's drawings and storytelling can reveal children's needs and perception of the disaster. For example, some children who are coping well may draw pictures of hurricanes but depict their family in a safe place. In contrast, children who have been traumatized may draw pictures of family members drowning or being hurt. Formal assessments with psychological instruments are not done in C³ARE due to the brevity of this intervention.

Refer—help families connect with their own social support network. Provide verbal and written referrals to formal support, specialized services, and resources. Helpful handouts include "Helping Children Cope with Disaster," which is available at www.fema.gov, and "Talking with and Helping Children and Youth after a Disaster or Traumatic Event," which is available at www.samhsa.gov/dtac.

Educate—teach children common responses to disasters, stress management strategies, and resiliency skills. See Tables 12.2 and 12.3 (Baggerly & Exum, 2008). Plans of action to meet immediate needs are also developed. Say: "Many children, but not all, have uncomfortable feelings or thoughts after something scary happens. Some children's bodies feel uncomfortable. It is okay if you do. Usually, it only lasts a short time. When you are upset, what do you usually do to feel better? I can teach you some new activities and games to help you." Play therapists can show children how to do "butterfly breathing" by putting their hands behind their head to slow down their heart rate. Then they can teach them another soothing activity of "butterfly hugs" by crossing arms over the chest and alternately patting arms. Children should be instructed to fold up any drawings of trauma reminders to contain in a safe space. Finally, play therapists can teach children to focus on the here and now through the 3-2-1 game of naming three things they can see above their eye level, three things they can hear, three things they can touch; then two things they can see, hear, and touch; and finally one thing they can see, hear, and touch.

After providing the C³ARE intervention to one family, play therapists inform them that they will be scheduling large group games later in the day to connect children from different families. Then play therapists scan the disaster relief area to determine the next family that may benefit from receiving C³ARE. It is important that play therapists are nonintrusive as they approach families. This nonintrusive approach can be accomplished by walking slowly toward people with a warm smile, standing by until eye contact is made, and then introducing self.

Kid's Corner.   When stabilization has been provided to all families who were open to the C³ARE intervention, play therapists can establish a "Kid's Corner" in an open area of the disaster relief area. The purpose of the Kid's Corner is not traditional play therapy but rather a play area where children can connect with others and enjoy familiar activities as a break from the chaos. A boundary for the Kid's Corner can be created by circling chairs around a large open area. Play therapists can organize and lay out expressive and nurturing toys such as cars, airplanes, dolls, medical kit, puppets, blocks, etc.; art materials such as crayons, markers, paper, clay, pipe cleaners, sand, miniatures, etc.; and games such as cards and checkers. Disaster relief experience has shown that a full range of aggressive release toys (i.e., guns, handcuffs, and Bobo) are not appropriate for this setting for two reasons (Baggerly, 2006b). First, the come and go nature of the Kid's Corner does not allow for adequate screening of participants. Some children may become overly aggressive when playing with aggressive release toys and may not respond to limits. Second, due to the open area, adult disaster survivors may be observing children and tend to view aggressive behavior in such a setting as threatening or disturbing. Therefore, it is best to adapt play therapy travel kits by removing all aggressive release toys.

When children enter the Kid's Corner, it is prudent to have their parents sign them in by logging the child's name, parent's name, cell phone number, and any medical concerns (i.e., allergies, diabetes, etc.). Providing the parent a claim check (i.e., number for the particular child) and placing a name tag on the child will help ensure safety for each child. When children play in the Kid's Corner, play therapists can track play

Table 12.2   Changes that Many Children Notice after a Disaster

Thoughts	*Feelings*
Confused	Scared
Can't think	Sad
Can't remember	Mad
Mean thoughts	Don't feel anything
Scary thoughts	Guilty
Always thinking about it	Embarrassed
Always remembering the bad part	Always stressed
Things We Do	*Body and Brain*
Sit alone	Staring off in the distance
Always looking around	Stomach ache
Yelling, hitting or fighting	Headache
Crying	Dizzy
Can't do school work	Sweaty for no reason
Not hungry or always hungry	Cold for no reason
Can't sleep or always sleep	Jumpy
Clumsy	Nightmares
Can't sit still	
Staying away from reminders of it	

God

Think God left
Confused about God
Mad at God
Don't want to pray, sing, or go to church/temple

behavior, reflect feelings, link children's play behavior, and set therapeutic limits as needed. However, it is not a formal group play therapy session.

Large Group Active Games.   After children have engaged in nondirective play in the Kid's Corner, play therapists can lead children in large group games. To introduce children to each other, it is helpful to begin with a name game. The Theraplay® Institute (2005) recommended a name game in which participants say "I am —" in various tones and voice pitches with other children responding "You are —" in the same manner three times. Since children in a disaster relief area have been confined inside for days typically, active gross motor games provide release of pent-up energy. One favorite game tends to be "Duck, Duck, Goose." In this game, children sit in a circle with one child walking outside of the circle, touching participants' heads and saying "duck." When the child says "goose," the one who was touched chases the other one around the circle. The first child tries to sit in the empty space before being tagged. If the child is tagged, then the child sits in the middle of the circle for three minutes. Other active game options include "Red Light, Green Light" (i.e., children run toward the finish line when the leader says "green light" and stop when the leader says "red light"); "Dance Freeze" (i.e., children dance and when the music is paused, they freeze); and relays of hopping, crawling backwards, three-legged races, etc. More active group games are described in Chapter 11.

Large Group Psycho-education.   Once children have had time to play and participate in active games, play therapists can lead children in a psycho-education session. The purpose of this psycho-education is to clarify disaster-related facts, normalize disaster-response symptoms, and increase positive coping strategies. To clarify facts, play therapists can create a puppet show in which a small puppet such as a puppy or rabbit pretends to be scared and asks a larger puppet such as a dog or owl questions of common misunderstandings about the disaster (Baggerly, 2006a).

RABBIT: I'm so scared about the hurricane coming that I keep running around in circles. Do you think the hurricane will be able to catch me?

OWL: Lots of little rabbits get scared and worried about the hurricane. The best way to be safe is to stay in the shelter with your family and be calm by cuddling with your family or playing games with other kids.

RABBIT: I had a bad dream that the hurricane destroyed my house. Maybe my dream will make it happen for real!

OWL: Little rabbit, dreams don't cause things to happen. Dreams just show us what we are worried about. Lots of people are worried about their houses.

RABBIT: But what if something bad happens to my house? Then what will me and my family do?

OWL: You are worried about the future. Right now, we are hoping for the best and doing our best to be calm right here, right now. Families who are kind and helpful to each other will be stronger no matter what happens.

An alternative to the puppet show is "news broadcast" (Kaduson & Schaefer, 2001). In this activity, the play therapist pretends to be a talk-show host and has children act as experts for mock questions that are phoned or emailed in. For example, the play therapist would say: "Welcome to K-N-O-W radio talk show. Today we are discussing the hurricane and I have with me several experts on the subject. Our first question is an email from Thomas who asks 'is the hurricane going to destroy or flood the whole city?' Experts, please answer this question for Thomas." The play therapist focuses on accurate points of the children and elaborates with other accurate information. For example, "I agree with the experts. Plus, the weather reporters have said only a small part of the city may have damage and lots of people are ready to help those who do have damage."

To normalize symptoms, play therapists can lead children in playing a game of charades in which children select a common symptom in the five realms discussed above and act it out for other children to guess. It is important for the play therapist to emphasize that not all children may notice these changes (i.e., symptoms) but those who have some will probably get better in a short time.

To increase positive coping, play therapists can also use charades to identify positive coping strategies in each of the five realms (see Table 12.2). After charades, play therapists can lead children in deep breathing by having children blow soap bubbles. Progressive muscle relaxation can be demonstrated by asking children to tense different muscle groups like a soldier and relax like a rag doll. Play therapists can end the group time with a positive affirmation cheer such as "When our family's in a bind, we'll be helpful, we'll be kind." Most of these play-based strategies for the immediate post-disaster phase are demonstrated in the video "Disaster mental health and crisis stabilization for children" (Baggerly, 2006a).

Short-term Adaptation Phase

In disaster recovery, the short-term adaptation phase usually occurs in the first few weeks and through the first year after a disaster. Since many children will continue to show typical symptoms and some will show more severe atypical symptoms, classroom-based or small group psycho-educational sessions are recommended to reduce symptoms and improve positive coping (La Greca & Silverman, 2009). There are several "empirically informed" manuals available online, such as *After the Storm* (La Greca, Sevin, & Sevin, 2005) and *Helping America Cope* (La Greca, Sevin, & Sevin, 2001) that can help children process the trauma and develop effective coping. However, these manual require an eighth-grade reading level and are not play-based interventions. Another intervention for this phase that has shown clinically and statistically significant reductions in PTSD and depression is Cognitive Behavioral Interventions after Trauma in Schools (CBITS) (Jaycox et al., 2010). However, research on CBITS was conducted with fourth graders and older children. For younger children, play is a developmentally appropriate approach (Landreth, 2012). Thus, Baggerly (2006b) and Drewes (2009) advise play therapists to blend cognitive behavioral approaches with play therapy strategies. The large group psycho-educational interventions described above can be implemented in a classroom or small group psycho-educational session.

Small Group Play Therapy

Children who are at risk for severe, ongoing atypical symptoms need more intensive intervention during this phase. Since research demonstrates that peer support is one of the biggest influences in disaster recovery (La Greca, Silverman, Lai, & Jaccard, 2010), small group play therapy is essential for children at risk for PTSD after a disaster. Play therapists select two to four children of similar gender and age. Small group play therapy is implemented via Trauma-Informed Child-Centered Play Therapy (TICCPT) (Baggerly, 2012). TICCPT integrates 30 minutes of standard group CCPT and cognitive behavioral psycho-educational activities (Baggerly, 2012).

CCPT.   During the 30 minutes of standard CCPT, play therapists track play behavior, reflect feelings and content, return responsibility, build self-esteem, facilitate understanding, and enlarge the meaning of disaster-related themes (Landreth, 2012). For example, I (Baggerly) led a small group play therapy session with a 6-year-old boy and his 7-year-old cousin who were evacuated from the New Orleans' Super Dome after Hurricane Katrina in 2005. During nondirected play, the boy stood on a chair and yelled "Oh no, the water is going to sweep me away." I reflected feelings with "You are really scared." He then jumped off the chair and pretended to drown. I facilitated understanding of his play by saying "you died like so many people did after the hurricane." His cousin ran over with a play medical kit and said "I'll save you." I reflected feelings with "you really want to rescue him." She pretended to bring her cousin back to life. I encouraged her with "you did it!" I also enlarged the meaning of her play behavior with "just like you, lots of people wanted to rescue others during the hurricane. They wish they had the power to do so because dying can be so sad and scary."

Small Group Psycho-educational Activities.   After 30 minutes of CCPT, play therapists inform children that it is time to do some other activities for 20 minutes. Then play therapists implement psycho-education activities to increase safety, manage hyperarousal, decrease intrusive symptoms, manage avoidance of disaster related to stimuli, decrease misattributions, and increase positive coping skills (Baggerly, 2012; Felix, Bond, & Shelby, 2006). These activities that are described below can be implemented sequentially with flexibility in selecting activities based on children's needs and developmental levels. Many of the play-based procedures described below are demonstrated in a video by Baggerly (2006a).

Safety Skills.   Safety skills are facilitated by asking children to play a game of identifying indicators that they are safe at the present time. This helps children learn to distinguish past fears with present situations. Children can draw a picture of a safe place and learn to hold that picture in their mind to develop a sense of psychological safety when they are physically safe. Play therapists can also help children to develop a safety plan and safety kit for future disasters.

Managing Hyperarousal.   To manage hyperarousal symptoms, play therapists can teach children self-soothing relaxation techniques to calm their bodies and deactivate their "fight or flight response" (Perry et al., 1995). Children can learn to take deep breaths through playful activities such as blowing pinwheels or pretending they are smelling a rose and then blowing out a candle. Play therapists can lead children through progressive muscle relaxation by asking them to tense muscle groups like a toy soldier and relax like a rag doll. Play therapists can teach children to focus on positive images by drawing happy places, engaging in mutual story telling that has a positive ending, or meditating on peaceful places (Baggerly, 2010).

Managing Intrusive Thoughts.   Play therapists teach children methods of managing intrusive thoughts of disaster-related events that are encoded in their implicit memory (Perry et al., 1995). One procedure is to "change the CD in your mind" by replacing negative thoughts with a predetermined positive song, story, or saying such as "I'm safe right now and I know it because I have …" Another procedure is thought stopping by drawing a stop sign on a popsicle stick and hitting the stick on a table while saying stop to a scary thought. Grounding activities such as rubbing stomach and rubbing hands together are also helpful procedures (Felix et al., 2006).

Managing Avoidance.   To help children manage avoidance of disaster-related stimuli, play therapists implement systematic desensitization procedures of pairing relaxation with a step-by-step hierarchy of exposure to the stimuli. For example, a child may be afraid to take a bath after a hurricane because of the association that occurred when the family sought shelter in the bathtub during the hurricane. In this example, the play therapist would teach the child to relax and then ask him to wipe his face with a wet wash cloth, gradually progressing to washing in a sink, then having the parent wash the child near the tub, and finally in the bathtub with small level of water, etc. (Baggerly, Green, Thorn, & Steele, 2007). Parents will need to be involved with these procedures and provide positive reinforcements for each accomplished step.

Managing Misattributions.   Due to their egocentric and concrete cognitions, some children may misattribute the cause of natural disasters to their bad dreams or someone's bad behavior. Play therapists should identify their misattributions and give accurate information. Procedures to correct misattributions include playing "garbage or treasure" by making a Q-sort of possible reasons for the disaster and asking children to sort them as garbage or treasure (i.e., untrue or true) (Felix et al., 2006). Play therapists can help children create a blame box to put drawings of who or what they blame for the disaster. Then the play therapist and children draw the correct reason together. Misattributions and accurate reasons can also be addressed through puppet shows or radio talk shows as described above.

Positive Coping.   Positive coping can be facilitated through bibliotherapy. The play therapist reads a children's story about trauma recovery such as *A Terrible Thing Happened* (Holmes, 2000) or *Brave Bart* (Shephard, 1998) in a soothing, calm voice. The play therapist can ask children to use puppets or toys to demonstrate how the book's characters responded to the disaster and ways they can cope. Then they can discuss how the characters' response was similar to, or different from, their own reactions and coping strategies.

Another bibliotherapy activity is for play therapists to read "Life Doesn't Frighten Me at All" by Maya Angelou (Green, Crenshaw, & Drewes, 2011). The play therapist asks the children to identify an image in the story that was prominent. Next, the play therapist asks them to draw a line down the middle of a piece of paper and create a scene of something they fear on the left side of the page. The play therapist observes in attentive silence. After the children are finished, the play therapist discusses the scene by discussing the symbols in the image: (a) "Did the story remind you of anything from your own life?" (b) "If you were in this image, how would you be feeling?" (c) "What story does this scene tell?" (d) "What occurred before/after this scene?" "If you could give this scene a title, what would it be?" Last, the play therapists ask the children to illustrate the concept of finally conquering their fear and anxiety so that it is manageable by illustrating it on the right side of the page.

An activity to personalize and internalize positive coping skills is called "The Coping Box" (Baggerly, 2007; Green, 2007; Felix et al., 2006). First, the play therapist obtains an old shoe box for each child and prompts them to place construction paper around the box and use a lid to cover it. Next, children look through magazines and cut out symbols or images that represent parts of their identity or something they can do to feel better during distress. The children glue the pictures on the box. The play therapist and the children write 10 coping strategies on 10 precut squares of construction paper. The

Table 12.3   Things Children Can Do To Feel Better After a Disaster

Thoughts	**Feelings**
Write things down or draw things	It is O.K. to cry
Do one thing at a time	It is O.K. to feel angry
Think about what you need	Say what you feel
Think of a plan	Talk about your feelings to your family and
Ask questions	friends
Think of a nice place to be and nice people	Laugh
Yell "stop" when you have bad thoughts	Remember happy feelings
Things We Do	**Body and Brain**
Play with others	Run and jump or ride a bike
Cuddle with family	Don't eat too many sweets
Help others	Drink water
Ask for help	Take deep, slow breaths
Have fun	Blow soap bubbles
Relax, relax, relax	Tense your muscles like a soldier and relax
Go outside	like a rag doll
Read books	
Sing and dance	
Draw	

God

Pray
Read spiritual books
Sing
Go to church or temple
Talk to your family or religious leader about God

children place the paper in their box, another child draws out a strategy, and the school counselor guides them in a role play to practice the coping strategy.

In the final group play therapy session, play therapists can reemphasize coping strategies by creating "A Coping Heart" (Baggerly, 2007; Green, 2007; Felix et al., 2006). The purpose of this intervention is to increase children's awareness of internalized coping strategies that can enhance future safety and development. The play therapist provides students with a piece of red construction paper with a predrawn large heart on it outlined in a dark color. The play therapist instructs the children to draw a line down the middle of the heart and a line across the middle of the heart so that there are roughly four equal sections. The children then consider activities they typically engage in to make themselves feel better when they are afraid or distressed. The children draw one of their coping activities in each of the four sections on the heart. After they are finished drawing, two small holes on the top edge of the heart are made by a hole puncher. The play therapist cuts a piece of yarn long enough to go around a child's neck and ties the heart around each child's neck. The play therapist instructs each child to tell others in the group what their coping strategies are and possibly role play them for the group. Last, play therapists remind children that they have the ability to protect their heart and keep it safe from harm by practicing and implementing these adaptive ways of coping with traumatic anxiety.

Long-term Recovery Phase

The last phase of disaster recovery is long-term recovery, which occurs from the end of the first year and beyond until children no longer exhibit symptoms and return to predisaster functioning or better. La Greca and Silverman (2009) stated the intervention with the strongest evidence during this phase is Trauma-Focused Cognitive Behavioral Therapy (TF-CBT; Cohen, Mannarino, & Deblinger, 2012). However, much of the evidence for TF-CBT is for older children. Thus, as in the short-term adaptation phase, play therapists are encouraged to integrate CBT with play therapy (Baggerly, 2012; Drewes, 2009). Details in this process are provided in Chapter 14.

Conclusion

Children are one of the most vulnerable populations during and after disasters. The United States National Commission on Children and Disasters recommended that mental health professionals such as play therapists be prepared to serve children after a disaster. Given the prevalence of natural and man-made disasters, an estimated 3 million U.S. children will be exposed to a disaster each year. Children's typical symptoms in the five realms of cognitive, emotional, behavioral, physical, and spiritual usually resolve in a short period of time. However, some children will have ongoing, severe atypical symptoms of depression, anxiety, and PTSD.

Play therapists must maintain disaster intervention principles such as deploying only when invited and maintaining a non-anxious presence throughout each phase of disaster recovery. During the immediate post-impact phase, play therapists can implement the Psychological First Aid C³ARE model of Check, Connect, Comfort, Access,

Refer, and Educate. They can also establish a Kid's Corner, facilitate large group active games, and large group psycho-education. During the short-term adaptation phase, play therapists can implement small group play therapy via TICCPT, which integrates 30 minutes of standard group CCPT and 20 minutes of cognitive behavioral psycho-educational activities. These activities will help children develop safety skills; manage hyperarousal, intrusive thoughts, avoidance, and misattributions; and increase positive coping.

Providing disaster response group play therapy can be more challenging than typical group play therapy because each child's development and sense of safety has been disrupted. Thus, play therapists must be vigilant in implementing their compassion fatigue resiliency plan of obtaining training, supervision, and self-care. Then play therapists can experience the rewards of disaster recovery group play therapy by helping children recover so that they will be resilient beings.

13 Group Play Therapy in Schools

Throughout this book, we highlight the rationale, significance, and process of group play therapy. Hence, the delivery of group play therapy in mental health settings can easily be seen as beneficial and necessary. School is a distinctive setting in which the facilitation of group play therapy may be impacted by unique features or obstacles within the environment. In schools, groups are commonly employed for educational purposes and economic efficiency (serving the greatest number with the fewest resources). The group model to mental health seemingly meets the format of school, yet the focus on play, child-led goals, and the primacy of an emotionally healthy path to academic success may be perceived as suspect in the school culture.

Schools typically employ mental health professionals for the purpose of helping children progress academically. In order for play therapists to justify their work in schools, it becomes imperative that they connect the intervention of play therapy to school success. Play therapy can be used to help a child feel safer, build positive school relationships, and learn with less internal distractions, all issues that will potentially lead to academic progress. When children accept themselves and develop positive self-regard, they will be more open to learning from others (Ray, 2011). Landreth (2012) claimed that the goal of play therapy in schools is to "help children get ready to profit from the learning experiences offered" (p. 148). In Axline's (1949) early studies on the positive link between play therapy and intelligence, she noted that play therapy allowed children to overcome emotional limitations that hindered expression of intelligence and release them to demonstrate full potential, leading to school achievement.

Early studies of CCPT measuring academic improvement suggested that play therapy helped to increase IQ scores and ability to learn in the classroom (Axline, 1949; Dulsky, 1942; Mundy, 1957; Shmukler & Naveh, 1984). Additionally, researchers (Newcomer & Morrison, 1974; Siegel, 1970) concluded that children with learning disabilities demonstrated significant improvement in motor functioning and learning difficulties as a result of participation in play therapy. Several recent studies have been conducted in elementary schools establishing a consistent pattern of incorporating play therapy in the school setting (Fall, Balvanz, Johnson, & Nelson, 1999; Fall, Navelski, & Welch, 2002; Garza & Bratton, 2005; Muro, Ray, Schottelkorb, Smith, & Blanco, 2006; Ray, 2007; Ray, Blanco, Sullivan, & Holliman, 2009; Ray, Schottelkorb, & Tsai, 2007; Schottelkorb & Ray, 2009; Schumann, 2010). These studies explored children's externalizing behaviors and relationships, specifically ADHD, aggression, and teacher–child relationships. Blanco and Ray (2011) conducted an experimental study of play therapy effect on first graders labeled as academically at-risk. They found that first graders significantly improved academic achievement following 16 sessions of play therapy over those who had not received play therapy, marking the first study in this century to link play therapy with academic achievement. Blanco, Ray, and Holliman (2012) followed the experimental group from the initial study and found that children continued to improve in academic achievement over the duration of 26 play therapy sessions. Although the Blanco and Ray (2011) study was conducted using individual play therapy, many school interventions have been conducted using group play therapy.

In a recent meta-analysis of play therapy research in the schools, Ray, Armstrong, Balkin, and Jayne (in review) analyzed results from 23 experimental studies from which they concluded that play therapy was statistically and qualitatively supported as an intervention in the schools. Effect sizes indicated that children participating in play therapy across studies improved problematic behaviors or characteristics at a statistically significant level when compared to their peers who received no intervention. Children demonstrated positive effects for internalizing and externalizing behavior, self-efficacy, academic, and other problems. When compared to alternative interventions, children participating in play therapy performed 0.20 standard deviations over their peers. The meta-analysis included the review of 13 studies utilizing individual play therapy and 10 studies utilizing group play therapy. There was no difference in outcome between individual and group modalities.

Types of Groups

There are typically two types of groups conducted in the school environment: Psycho-educational groups and counseling groups (Cobia & Henderson, 2007). Psycho-educational groups, often referred to as guidance in schools, focus on learning and prevention. They address specific problems or potential problems, such as preventing test anxiety or developing communication skills. Psycho-educational groups that use play as a mechanism to make teaching points or reach educational objectives would most closely align to a cognitive-behavioral approach to group play therapy. They can also be delivered to small or large groups of children. Counseling groups are offered to small groups of children in the school in order to address a problem or developmental issues. They respond to the intrapersonal and interpersonal needs of children. Counseling groups delivered in a group play therapy modality use play as the main communication tool for members of the group. Play therapy counseling groups can be facilitated from any of the theoretical orientations to play therapy.

Because there are multiple resources available for the implementation of psycho-educational groups utilizing play in the schools (e.g., Ashby et al., 2008; Parsons, 2007; Reddy, 2012), this chapter will focus mostly on the implementation of play therapy through counseling groups. Group play therapy in schools serves to address the interpersonal issues that affect or impede academic progress. The emphasis is on providing a group experience in which children can communicate through their language of play and interact with peers in a natural setting. Group is established so that children are faced with peer interaction and encouraged to develop the interpersonal skills to facilitate such interaction. Play structures such as nondirective play, child-centered play, sandtray, and expressive arts are most conducive to support focus on natural interpersonal interaction and skills.

Case Example

In this example, eight children had been referred to the school counselor from kindergarten and three from first grade for having social skill problems and being disruptive in class. Because it was October and the kindergartners were still new to the school structure, the counselor utilized a psycho-educational group curriculum to address how to make friends. She implemented the curriculum over 6 weeks with 30-minute sessions per week. She also worked individually with the teacher to help manage behavioral problems in the classroom. Because the referred first graders had shown problems since the previous year and those problems appeared to be worsening, the counselor chose to conduct a child-centered play therapy group for eight sessions. The three children were all boys, came from different home circumstances, but demonstrated interpersonal problems.

Group Members

Miguel. Miguel was 6 years old, Latino, and lived in a home where Spanish was the only language spoken. Miguel spoke English and Spanish fluently. Miguel lived with both of his biological parents who both worked outside the home in the evening. Miguel had two older adolescent brothers who were in charge of him in the evenings. Miguel engaged in frequent fights on the playground and interpreted many peer interactions throughout the day as aggression toward him.

Cody. Cody was Caucasian, spoke English only, and was 6 years old. He lived with a single mother and had never known his dad. Cody demonstrated odd behaviors at school, such as constantly talking to himself, picking at his skin, and speaking in a loud, monotone voice. He had no friends at school and his mother reported that he had no friends at home. He had difficulty connecting with the teacher or other school adults and always seemed "in his own world."

David. David was Latino but only spoke English, and he just turned 7 years old. He lived with his biological mother, who gave birth to David when she was 15 years old, and his new stepdad who had just started living with David and his mother in the past year. David was physically larger than most of his classmates. Although he did not initiate hitting others, he used his size and threats to intimidate others into giving him what he wanted by grabbing or shoving. Many of the children were scared of David and avoided him. He had also cursed at his teacher on multiple occasions.

Group Screening

The school counselor met with each of the boys individually in a play therapy session to assess their appropriateness for group. She decided that none of the boys seemed too aggressive or interpersonally limited to benefit from group play therapy. She also determined that the personality of the boys might serve to help them relate to one another.

Two of the boys, Miguel and Cody, were in the same classroom and David was in the classroom across the hall. All of the boys knew each other through Specials classes (art, music, P.E.) and recess. Miguel and David had played together on the playground and had one previous loud argument but had not fought. Due to Cody's isolating behaviors, he had not played with Miguel or David previously. The counselor worked out a schedule with the teachers in which the group would take place for 30 minutes twice a week for 4 weeks. The group met during the small group educational time in class when children worked at tables independently.

Beginning Stage

Because the counselor was delivering group play therapy from a child-centered approach, the playroom included a large open space with multiple toys and play materials on shelves, a puppet theater, and a sand box. As the children entered the room, the counselor said: "In here is the playroom, you can play with the toys in lots of the ways you like." The boys fanned out to different parts of the room.

CODY [goes to far corner of room and picks up a snake, and directs his comment to no one in particular, looking at the wall]: This is my snake George and he loves me.

MIGUEL [picks up gun and points at therapist]: Look at this. Bang! Bang!

DAVID [first goes to cars but looks at Miguel when he picks up gun, crosses room, and stands right beside Miguel towering over him]: Let me see.

Miguel, looking intimidated, gives gun over to David.

COUNSELOR: You guys are pretty excited about being in here. Really checking things out.

Cody continues to stay in the corner with the snake, folding it around him, and talking to it. Miguel then finds the foam sword, picks it up, and starts to swish it back and forth.

DAVID [still holding gun, heads over to Miguel]: Let me see it.

MIGUEL [to David]: You point the gun at me; I'll fight you with the sword.

DAVID [moves even closer to Miguel]: No, give me the sword. I'll give you the gun.

Miguel reluctantly gives David the sword but David does not give Miguel the gun.

MIGUEL [looks at the counselor]: Hey! You said I could have the gun.

COUNSELOR: Miguel you're mad. You think David should have given you the gun.

MIGUEL: Yeah, that's not fair. He said he would give me the gun.

COUNSELOR: And you think I should do something about it. [As David continues to play with the gun and sword]. And David, you think it's okay to keep both of them and not give one to Miguel.

David ignores both Miguel and the counselor. Miguel mutters a curse word in Spanish under his breath and goes over to Cody's side of the room. He picks up a dragon and tries to have the dragon interact with Cody's snake. Cody turns his back to Miguel. Miguel moves over to the dress-up clothes and starts to go through them.

This initial stage involves several dynamics between children and between children and counselor. The therapist is attempting to allow many interactions to occur without intervention in order to assess the children's normal responses to peer interaction. In this scenario, some dynamics were predictable such as Cody's isolating behavior or David's intimidating behavior. But some dynamics were less predictable, such as Miguel's decision to acquiesce to David. The therapist noted that Miguel seemed to respond to the hierarchy of physical power displayed by David. He did not seem to know how to advocate or negotiate for himself. Another dynamic noted by the therapist was the children's nonverbal interactions. Although Cody did not interact with the other children, he occasionally looked around to see what they were doing. After Cody rejected Miguel's attempt to play with him, Cody glanced more frequently at Miguel for the rest of the session. After David and Miguel's interaction, David also occasionally looked around to see what Miguel was doing. Another significant observation was that Miguel demonstrated the most social hunger of the three. He seemed to have a need to connect with both children and the counselor, possibly indicating that he will be the catalyst for future group interactions.

Middle Stage

As sessions progressed, Miguel and David continued to want to play with the same materials. In order to entice David to play, Miguel often gave in to what David wanted. Additionally, Cody began to move closer to where David and Miguel played. Although he acted as if he were playing with his snake exclusively, he would sometimes direct the snake's comments to Miguel and David. The following excerpt is from the fourth session:

DAVID [to Miguel]: I'm the police and you're the bad guy. You just stole something. I'm going to tie you up.

MIGUEL [as David moves toward him to tie him with rope, he steps back]: No.

DAVID [keeps moving toward Miguel]: But you're the bad guy, you have to be tied up. C'mon.

COUNSELOR: David, you really want to tie up Miguel, but Miguel, you really don't want to be tied up.

MIGUEL: No, I don't want to.

CODY [who has moved closer to the action sees Miguel's stress, holds the snake out]: You can tie up George. He's been bad.

MIGUEL: Yeah, let's make George the bad guy.

COUNSELOR: Cody, you thought of another way to work it out.

DAVID: No, he has to be real. He has to be tied up to the chair.

MIGUEL: We can tie George up to the chair.

CODY: But don't hurt him.

COUNSELOR: Cody, you're worried about George.

MIGUEL: No, we won't hurt him.

COUNSELOR: Miguel, you'll make sure George doesn't get hurt.

DAVID [directed at the snake]: Okay, George, you've been a real bad guy. Time for jail.

COUNSELOR: David, you decided this just might work.

In this scenario, each child is being confronted with the peer interactions that have caused them distress in the past. Previously, they have been unable to be creative or successful in their efforts to negotiate for their needs, thus they moved to less effective methods, such as aggression or withdrawal. They are now able to practice new coping skills to get their needs met. Miguel wants to play but does not feel strong enough to win a battle against David. Cody wants to be a part of the group but does not know how to do that directly. And David wants his way but does not know how to get his needs met unless he is the aggressor or decider. This was their first interaction in which all three creatively sought new solutions and sacrificed some of their needs for needs of another. This pattern continued during the middle stage of the group with the boys becoming more creative and frequent in their interactions.

Ending Stage

Because of the time limitations imposed by school structure, timing of termination was artificially decided prior to the beginning of group. During the middle stage, the boys engaged in frequent and effective interpersonal problem-solving. As the boys moved toward the end of therapy, new dynamics started to emerge. At the beginning of the seventh session, the counselor said: "Guys, I just wanted to remind you that we have today and one more time before our group ends. Thursday will be our last time for play group."

MIGUEL: Awww, man. Why? Can't we come back next week?

COUNSELOR: You're really disappointed. You want group to keep going.

DAVID: Yeah, c'mon, can't we? We all want to. Cody, right?

CODY [playing with the stuffed animals]: Huh?

DAVID: Tell Ms. Brown that you want to keep coming.

CODY [moves toward others]: Yes, I want to keep coming.

COUNSELOR: I can see that you guys really like coming and you want to keep coming.

All three boys stand in front of counselor, pleading "yeah, please, please." "Can we just keeping coming for two more weeks?" "Please Ms. Brown, please?"

COUNSELOR: You really want me to know how important this is to you. And it's hard to say good-bye to the play group.

MIGUEL: We can still play at recess.

COUNSELOR: Miguel, you thought of a whole other way for you guys to play together.

MIGUEL: Yeah, Cody and I play at group time in Ms. Smith's class.

CODY [smiles]: Yeah.

COUNSELOR: So, there's a whole other time you can find to play together.

DAVID: Miguel and me played soccer at recess. I picked Miguel for my team.

MIGUEL [looking at David]: I'm going to pick you for my team next time. Anthony wanted me to pick him but I'm picking you.

DAVID: Anthony plays really good. He's the best kicker. You should pick him.

MIGUEL: Okay, I'll pick you second.

As the boys enter this final stage of therapy, there are two significant dynamics taking place. The first is the cohesion displayed among the group members. Each member is engaged in what is taking place and desires to interact. Each member is cognizant of the other and attempting to be aware of the others' needs. The second dynamic is the transfer of focus and skills from inside the group to outside the group. The boys identified how they are taking their awareness and skills and using them outside of the playroom. The result of this transfer for these boys was improved interpersonal functioning within the classroom and with peers.

Evaluation of Group

Because the boys were referred by teachers and problems seemed most prevalent at school, the counselor conducted evaluation of the group through the teachers. Prior to the beginning of group, the counselor asked the teachers to fill out a quick behavioral assessment on each of the boys. The counselor also talked to the teachers about the boys, listing their concerns and explaining how group play therapy will address those concerns. In the middle stage, the counselor checked in with the teachers to see if they had noticed any changes. Miguel and Cody's teacher reported that she had seen Miguel and Cody talking during class, an interaction that had not taken place previously. In order to talk to Miguel, Cody had lowered the volume of his voice and even had more feeling inflection in his tone. She said that Miguel was still likely to get upset about peer interactions that did not go his way but he had not initiated any fights recently. David's teacher reported that she noticed he was keeping a greater physical distance from his peers and was waiting his turn in line throughout the day. At the ending of the group, the counselor met with each teacher who reported substantial improvements in the behavior of all three boys. On post-assessments given by the counselor, scores also indicated improvement.

Considerations for Application of Group Play Therapy in Schools

Structure

Structural elements of group play therapy are often shaped by the school environment. Length of intervention, length of sessions, timing of sessions, and playroom space are influenced by school schedules, building resources, and staff. Group play therapy can be especially difficult to maneuver logistically in order to accommodate the simultaneous needs and school demands of multiple children.

Length of Intervention

As emphasized earlier, group play therapy in schools serves the academic purpose of school. All school counseling interventions are designed to support the educational goals of the school and individual students. Hence, counseling is typically offered in short-term interventions in order to avoid as many academic scheduling conflicts as possible. Conflicts include the removal of children from academic lessons in the classroom in order to deliver group play therapy. Group play therapy in schools needs to be conceived as a short-term process to increase the child's motivation and engagement in the classroom. Because of this focus, the length of group play therapy is determined prior to the beginning of the group. In the case example, we presented a group play therapy model that would take place twice a week for 4 weeks. Such a model allows for intensive counseling but for a short length of time. The intervention can be delivered in consideration of standardized testing, i.e., offering group play therapy for the month of October if standardized testing takes place in the spring. The counselor may consult with the teacher about particular units of study so that the teacher and counselor work in collaboration regarding timing of the intervention.

School counseling interventions are usually shorter than 8–10 weeks. If problems are still significant, a school mental health professional is encouraged to refer the child to an outside counselor. Many mental health professionals have difficulty with this short-term perspective and will need to adjust their views to be successful in the school setting.

Length of Sessions

The length of sessions is also impacted by the focus on short-term intervention and need to maintain the child's exposure to academics. Whereas many private therapists will hold group play therapy sessions for 45 minutes up to an hour and half, school sessions typically last for approximately 30 minutes. Shorter sessions are needed to reduce the amount of time the child is removed from the classroom. If a school or teacher is supportive of longer sessions, the counselor would be encouraged to lengthen sessions to a minimum of 45 minutes. Because length of sessions and length of intervention are shortened in the school setting, play therapy groups operate as closed groups so that safety between members and therapists can be established as quickly as possible. In a closed group, members in the group remain the same throughout the intervention.

Timing of Sessions

Just as teachers and administrators are concerned about the child's absence from academic lessons, children are concerned about absence from the more fun aspects of school, such as recess or physical education. The school play therapist needs to balance the school's academic concerns with the child's needs when planning for group play therapy. Group play therapy sessions are less successful to sustain when scheduled during recess. Children will delay participation or spend their time during therapy distracted by thoughts of outside play. Also, with limited amounts of free play offered to most school children, the play therapist values the mental health benefits of outside play and physical movement. Group play therapy should be scheduled with careful attention to the effects of academic or nonacademic absences.

Space and Play Materials

Although group play therapy is ideally practiced in a spacious playroom with an adequate number of toys, play therapy can be effective in different sizes of rooms. Play therapists in schools may be limited by room access or materials. Essential features of a playroom include shelves for placing toys above the floor, allowing more room for movement, and at least some space for free movement. Group play especially requires the need for enough room for children to move so that they are not forced into intruding upon others' space.

Optimal features in a playroom for a group include access to water through a sink, non-carpeted floors, and durable wall paint. Yet, school play therapists can successfully facilitate group play in a conference room, bookroom, behind a cafeteria stage, or in a portable building. Counselors in schools are often assigned offices, some small and some large. In small spaces, school counselors should be creative with room placement. Shelves can be used to place toys within reach of children and still provide floor space. Desk room might be minimized to create more free space in the office. A conference table might double as a craft table. If a school counselor is one of the fortunate few who is assigned a classroom, dividers/shelves can be used to divide parts of the room (Ray, 2011). One part of the room should be partitioned large enough to conduct group play therapy.

A portable playroom can be developed to allow school play therapists to operate out of most spaces. Toys can be stored in large tote bags or large plastic bins, preferably on wheels. For sessions, play therapists lay out toys in an organized way prior to the session. The group play therapist seeks to provide as much consistency as possible regarding meeting place and materials. Another consideration for group play therapy in the schools is confidentiality. Because of the active nature of group play therapy, sessions are likely to be louder than average individual sessions. The play therapist takes extra precautions to ensure confidentiality by working with administrators to address any threats to confidentiality. At times, the play therapist may address volume with children so they realize the effect of their vocalizations, often helpful to children who are struggling with social skills.

Play materials in the schools may need special consideration. Unlike private practice settings where therapists can select the ages of children they serve or modify their room and materials to meet developmental needs of children at different ages, school play therapists must operate with materials that meet the developmental needs of those between 5 and 12 years old. Materials in the room need to be functional for a broad range of chronological differences. Ray (2011) recommended organizing materials into age groups and scheduling play therapy accordingly. Some craft materials may be placed in locked cabinets that are open on Mondays and Tuesdays when the play therapist sees groups of fourth and fifth graders and some toy carts are rolled out on Wednesdays and Thursdays when the play therapist sees groups of kindergarten and first graders. Versatility of space and materials is essential to effective group play therapy in schools.

Teachers and Administrators

Teachers and administrators are key stakeholders in the educational lives of children. Successful facilitation of group play therapy is dependent on the support and collaboration of school staff. Referral to play therapy is conducted by teachers who are usually the first adults to notice that a child is in need of mental health intervention. Once a referral is made, the play therapist works with school staff to implement group play therapy, requiring the support of teachers and administrators. Similar to the process of gaining support for individual play therapy, play therapists educate school staff about the process of group play therapy, including the rationale, benefits, and procedures. Ray (2011) presented eight methods to gain support for a play therapy program in schools including:

- Present the basics of play therapy, including how it benefits the teacher and class-room overall, at staff development workshops.
- Present referral procedures and walk teachers through the process of how the play therapist will be handling individual cases of students.
- Present toys used in the playroom, allowing teachers and administrators to have a concrete idea of what takes place in play therapy.
- Provide teachers and administrators with evaluation data to support the play therapy program, including data collected from teachers about changes in children.
- Integrate play into everyday school interactions. Offer a 5–10-minute group play activity at monthly meetings. When teachers and administrators experience play at this level, they may be able to appreciate the implementation of a play therapy program for children.
- Provide play materials accessible to school staff such as a small sandtray or hand toys for use when teachers or administrators visit the counselor's office.
- Individually communicate with teachers about their concerns about children. Respond to these concerns by addressing through action (offering interventions to child).
- Sustain continued consultation with teachers about individual children, keeping them updated, within the limitations of confidentiality, about children's participation in counseling.

Evaluation

Schools operate from an orientation of accountability. Evidence-based interventions and collection of data regarding implemented interventions are suggested routes to meeting the criteria for accountability. When working to implement group play therapy in the schools, counselors should provide administrators with research to support the effectiveness of group play therapy. Presenting research conducted on play therapy in the schools will promote the support of administrators for group play therapy as an academic intervention. Summaries provided at the beginning of this chapter regarding the link between play therapy and academic achievement, as well as research provided at the end of this book supporting the positive effects of group play therapy, provide evidence that group play therapy is a viable intervention for schools.

Evaluation plans are critical to securing support for group play therapy work in the schools. Schools are under pressure to provide evidence, not only for the support of a school mental health intervention, but more importantly for the use of the intervention as contributing to school goals. Play therapists can connect their work to school vision by developing evaluation plans to that end (Ray, 2011). Evaluation methods that are utilized in schools may include grades, teacher reports, standardized testing, discipline referrals, and psychological/behavioral testing. For group play therapy, play therapists might consider social skills measures that are collected prior to the beginning of therapy and directly after termination. If play therapists are limited in their access to formal assessments, they might create short questionnaires of five to ten items related to presenting problems of children referred for group play therapy. Even informal assessment can help support a play therapy program.

Conclusion

Group play therapy in schools involves special considerations beyond its implementation in agency or private practice settings. When the primary goal for play therapy in the schools is academic progress, the path to mental health or healing may become less clear. The selection of children to participate in group is influenced by teacher, parent, or self-referral, as well as extent of presenting problem. The particularly difficult task of balancing educational exposure with mental health and interpersonal functioning can be daunting for even the most experienced play therapists. The play therapist benefits from operating within an educational framework and initiating efforts to gain the collaboration of school stakeholders. The benefits of offering group play therapy in schools to children who are interpersonally impaired far outweigh the limitations placed on the process by educational requirements.

14   Healing Bereavement and Loss

Bereavement is a period of mourning and grief that occurs after the death of a beloved person or animal. Bereavement is experienced by millions of U.S. children every year. The death of a parent impacts approximately 3.7 million of the 74 million U.S. children. "In the United States, one out of every twenty children lives with either one or no parent because of death" (Massat, Moses, & Ornstein, 2008, p. 82). Children grieving the death of a sibling, child family member, or friend is estimated in the hundreds of thousands per year. In 2010, approximately 42,700 U.S. children died, including nearly 24,600 under 1 year; 4,300 aged 1 to 4 years; 2,300 aged 5 to 9; over 2,900 aged 10 to 14; and 10,900 aged 15 to 19 (Center for Disease Control, 2011).

Loss of relationship with a person, animal, or place (i.e., country, home, school) can also cause grief. Children's grief due to loss of relationships may occur for numerous reasons, including parent's divorce, entering foster care, parent's military deployment, moving with family, having a significant adult move away, or having pets that are missing or given away. In 2009, there were 1.1 million U.S. children whose parents divorced (Elliot & Simmons, 2011). In 2011, there were 252,320 U.S. children who entered foster care and thus lost their daily relationship with a significant parent or guardian (U.S. Department of Health and Human Services, 2012). An organization called Our Military Kids (2013) reported an estimated 58,000 U.S. children aged 3 to 18 had a parent with a military deployment and another 54,000 had a parent recovering from severe injury sustained during service. According to the 2010 U.S. Census, the number of families with children who moved within the year was 4.8 million. Based on these data, millions of U.S. children have experienced a significant loss in the last year and many are likely to be experiencing grief.

Given the enormous prevalence of children who experience bereavement and loss every year, play therapists need to increase their competence with this population of children. Fearnley (2010) stated:

> The needs of children who are experiencing the death of a parent or caregiver or who have been bereaved are often overlooked and not addressed as urgently or as directly as they should be. It has been argued that two associated reasons for this serious omission are a lack of training and ongoing professional development and professionals' perceptions of their own lack of competence to communicate with this emotionally challenging community of children.
>
> (p. 458)

The purpose of this chapter is to prepare play therapists to serve grieving children by discussing: (a) the impact of bereavement and loss on children; (b) preparation for group play therapy with bereaved children; and (c) Trauma-Informed Child-Centered Group Play Therapy procedures.

Impact of Bereavement and Loss on Children

Common Grief Symptoms in Children

Like children who have experienced disasters, children who have experienced a loved one's death or loss may show symptoms in five realms (see Chapter 12). In the cognitive realm, children may search for answers, be confused, hold irrational beliefs, blame self, lack trust in others, be inattentive in academics, and have intrusive memories or nightmares (Cohen, Mannarino, & Deblinger, 2006; Webb, 2007). In the affective realm, children may experience fear, depression, anger, anxiety, worry about wellbeing of loved ones, and display affective dysregulation. In the physical realm, children may have weight changes, stomach aches, headaches, sleeplessness, thumb sucking, or enuresis. In the behavioral realm, children may have clinginess due to separation anxiety, school refusal, hyperactivity, aggression, fights with peers or family members, and avoidance of reminders of the deceased person or animal. In the spiritual realm, children may have doubts about God, abandon spiritual rituals such as prayers or attending religious services, have a diminished sense of the future, and hold a "self-fulfilling prophecy" (e.g., "I'll die in a car accident when I'm 35 like my mom did") (Cohen et al., 2006; Webb, 2007).

In addition to these symptoms, children may also maintain a relationship with the deceased in a fantasized way (Schoen et al., 2004). Goldman (2006) stated a bereaved child may "emulate the conduct of the deceased, consistently wear something of the loved one, constantly tell their story, and speak of the loved one in the present" (p. 569). Although maintaining a relationship with the deceased can be culturally appropriate (i.e., prayer, shrine, burning candles, etc.), it is only considered unhealthy if it prevents the child from social or emotional functioning in his or her environment.

As indicated in this long list of possible symptoms, it is important to note that children may not always display their grief in the form of sadness. For example, one child may have unspoken anxiety about a surviving parent's wellbeing, while another child may have anger that is displaced on the soccer field and still another child may seem relatively happy most of the time with only a few moments of upset. Thus, just because a child is not sad or crying does not mean the child is not grieving.

Variables Influencing Children's Grief Response

Children's experience and expression of bereavement vary based on developmental level due to different cognitive understandings of death's irreversibility, finality, inevitability, and causality (Willis, 2002). Children 2–5 years old do not understand the permanence of death and may believe the person has moved away (Willis, 2002). Due to their magical thinking, preschool children may even believe the deceased will come back to life. "Maybe if I am a good girl and clean my room then grandma will come back because she said she didn't want to be in a messy room." Preschoolers' limited concepts of time and space can contribute to young children's belief that something they did near the time of death caused the death. For example, a 4-year-old may say "I was mad at grandma for putting me in time out and yelled at her. She said that hurt her. The next day she died from a heart attack. I made her die." After a death, preschoolers' play behaviors tend to be about reuniting with the deceased, who magically comes back to life (Le Vieux, 1999).

Children 6–9 years old understand that death is irreversible but may believe that it can be avoided (Willis, 2002). Hence, they can become preoccupied and anxious about the wellbeing of loved ones (Le Vieux, 1999). Some school-aged children may also have fears that they caused the death but tend not to verbalize these fears. Attribution statements such as "God needed grandma in heaven" may be misunderstood and result in school-aged children quietly holding anger at God. In an attempt to avoid feeling overwhelmed by emotional pain, school-aged children may be hyperactive, silly, noncompliant, or pretend that things are just normal. Play themes tend to be about protecting family members, friends, and others from peril and/or burying representative objects.

Children 9–12 years old understand that death is permanent and inevitable (Willis, 2002). In an effort to be like their peers, they may be self-conscious and keep emotions inside. This internalized grief may result in extreme moodiness, depression, anxiety, and psychosomatic symptoms (e.g., headache, stomach ache). Play therapy, sandplay, and expressive arts are particularly helpful as nonverbal symbolic processing of events circumvents reluctance and embarrassment. For example, these children may use miniature animals to construct elaborate funeral processions in the sandtray.

Children's grief symptoms are also impacted by numerous risk and resiliency factors. Risk factors that predict children will have more symptoms include prior trauma exposure, female gender, close relationship to the deceased, witnessing the death, and stressful events following the death (e.g., separation from other family members, parental distress, financial difficulties) (Cohen et al., 2006; Haine, Ayers, Sandler, & Wolchik, 2008; Webb, 2007). Resiliency factors that predict children will have fewer symptoms include open communication, coping skills, parental warmth, and other external sources of support (Cohen, Mannarino, & Deblinger, 2006; Haine et al., 2008; Webb, 2007).

Based on these variables, children's grief responses and symptoms range in intensity, frequency, duration, and complexity. Symptoms may resolve within weeks or months or continue for over a year. Symptoms may also surface briefly during reminders (i.e., funerals, birthdays, and death anniversary) or randomly outside of a context (i.e., while playing with friends, watching T.V., or sitting in a classroom). Since there is no one right way or time to grieve, adults should never impose a grief response or timeline on children. Rather, adults should convey that "every child grieves in different ways at different times so whatever you feel and whenever you feel it is O.K. I am here to help when you need me."

Uncomplicated Grief vs. Complicated Grief

Distinguishing uncomplicated grief from complicated grief or childhood traumatic grief will help parents and play therapists determine the level of needed intervention (Cohen et al., 2006). Uncomplicated grief is the typical process of grieving the loss of an important relationship without having it result in Major Depressive Disorder (MDD). Usually, MDD is not diagnosed until after 2 months after the death of a loved one, unless the person has:

> Feelings of guilt other than actions taken or not taken by the survivor at the time of death
>
> Thoughts of death other than feelings he or she would be better off dead or should have died with the deceased person
>
> Morbid preoccupation with worthlessness
>
> Sluggishness or hesitant and confused speech
>
> Prolonged and marked difficulty in carrying out the activities of day-to-day living
>
> Hallucinations other than thinking he or she hears the voice of or sees the deceased person.
>
> (APA, 2000, p. 741)

Uncomplicated grief in children is no longer conceptualized as progression through Kübler-Ross's five stages of grief (i.e., denial, anger, bargaining, depression, and acceptance). Rather, current bereavement researchers conceptualize uncomplicated grief in children as the accomplishment of certain tasks (Cohen et al., 2006). According to Baker, Sedney, and Gross (1992), uncomplicated grief in children would occur by accomplishing the following tasks during three phases.

> Early Phase:
> Understanding the fact that someone has died and the implications of this fact.
> The children focus on the protection of themselves and their families.
> Middle Phase:
> Accepting and emotionally acknowledging the reality (and permanency) of the loss.
> Exploring and reevaluating the relationship to the lost loved one.
> Late Phase:
> The child needs to invest in a new relationship with others.
> The child must be able to internalize the lost relationship with the deceased person that will be there for him/her over time.
> The child will be able to return to their previous developmental level and activities.
> The child will be able to cope with the return of painful affect at different times in their developmental transitional periods.
>
> (Kirwin & Hamrin, 2005, p. 73)

TEAR is a helpful acronym that summarizes these tasks (Life Center of the Suncoast, 2005):

T = To accept the reality of the loss
E = Experience the pain of the loss
A = Adjust to the new environment without the loss
R = Reinvest in the new reality

In contrast to uncomplicated grief, complicated grief, also called childhood traumatic grief in children, occurs when there are unresolved grief and PTSD symptoms as well as possible depressive symptoms (Cohen et al., 2006). Unresolved grief manifests as yearning and searching for the deceased as well as difficulty accepting the death. "The PTSD symptoms include intrusive/preoccupying thoughts; dreams or memories about the traumatic death and/or the deceased; avoidance of reminders of the deceased; and/or the trauma reminders related to the death; emotional numbness or detachment; and hyperarousal symptoms, including anger or bitterness related to the death" (Cohen et al., 2006, p. 17). Children who have complicated, childhood traumatic grief first need intensive intervention for the trauma and then intervention for the grief to mitigate serious long-term mental health problems such as depression, substance abuse, and borderline personality disorder.

Preparation for Bereavement Work

Personal Preparation

Personal reflection on one's view of death is needed to prevent counter-transference and compassion fatigue within play therapists. This reflection begins with play therapists remembering their own experience with death or loss of a loved one. Although this task may be uncomfortable or painful, it may reveal a need to fully embrace an existential reality of death. In an article entitled *Freedom and Death*, Baker (2005) writes "To deny death is to impose limitations on our life and our culture, creating 'reality' based on short-term vision and immediate gratification which can leave us spiritually bankrupt" (p. 1). Hence, play therapists are encouraged to hold a positive perspective on death. Baker stated "Close encounters with death may awaken us deeply to our spiritual life purpose and to an appreciation for loving unconditionally" (p. 1). If play therapists discover an inability to maintain a positive view of death, then they are advised to seek counseling and supervision before treating children who are grieving.

Caregiver Interview

Interviewing the caregiver provides a context for understanding children's experiences, perceptions, prior functioning level, current needs, and potential play behaviors. For example, a child who witnessed a death may have different self-talk (e.g., "I should have stopped him from running into the street") compared to a child who learned of the death hours later (e.g., "I wish I was there but I was already at school"). Interacting with caregivers also provides helpful clues on the caregiver's level of coping. Some caregivers may be appropriately tearful but indicate that they are also receiving counseling and family support. Yet, other caregivers may be so overwhelmed that they have difficulty functioning on a day-to-day basis. Since children take their coping cues from caregivers, it is prudent to refer caregivers who are not coping well to seek their own counseling. This will help them to be more emotionally available for their children.

Assessment

Assessment of children can be helpful in determining the severity of symptoms and specific problem areas such as nightmares, avoidance of trauma reminders, inaccurate beliefs, etc. Assessments also serve as a pretest and posttest to determine treatment efficacy. Some common assessments for children who have experienced death and loss are:

> *UCLA PTSD Index for DSM-IV* (Pynoos et al., 1998)
>
> *Children's PTSD Inventory* (Saigh, 2004)
>
> *Trauma Symptom Checklist for Young Children* (Briere, 2005)
>
> *Child and Adolescent Needs and Strengths-Trauma Exposure and Adaptation* (Lyons, Griffin, Fazio, & Lyons, 1999)
>
> *Revised Manifest Anxiety Scale* (Reynolds & Richmond, 1985)
>
> *Children's Depression Inventory* (Kovacs, 1982).

Group Composition

As discussed in previous chapters, general guidelines for group composition include: (a) participants who are on the same developmental level, typically within 2 years of age; (b) same gender after third grade; and (c) committed to attending sessions on a regular basis. Le Vieux (1999) also recommended combining grieving children whose loved one died by various causes such as illness, accidents, homicide, or suicide. This composition allows children to understand the many shapes and forms of death, learn sensitivity to various situations, and offer different perspectives.

Trauma-Informed Child-Centered Group Play Therapy

One prominent and promising treatment modality that is commonly used by child therapists to improve young children's mental health is child-centered play therapy (CCPT) (Baggerly, Ray, & Bratton, 2010; Landreth, 2012). CCPT is based primarily on the child's natural language of play, which is developmentally appropriate for young children, especially if they are grieving. CCPT has been shown to improve the mental health of children who were homeless (Baggerly, 2004); were witnesses of domestic violence (Tyndall-Lind et al., 2001); had experienced natural disasters (Shen, 2002); and were refugees (Schottelkorb, Doumas, & Garcia, 2012).

Building on the success of CCPT, Baggerly (2012) recommends Trauma-Informed Child-Centered Play Therapy (TICCPT) as a treatment for children who have experienced trauma such as death or loss of a loved one. TICCPT is an evidence-informed approach that infuses trauma awareness, knowledge, and skills into CCPT (Landreth, 2012) by adding 15–25 minutes of psycho-education. The psycho-education entails lower brain neuro-developmental activities (e.g., Theraplay®; Booth & Jernberg, 2010) as well as evidence-based cognitive behavioral activities (e.g., Trauma-Focused Cognitive Behavior Therapy [TF-CBT]; Cohen et al., 2006). Parent consultation is provided but parents are not required to participate in every session.

TICCPT fulfills three fundamental components of trauma recovery identified by Judith Herman (1992): "(1) establishing safety, (2) restorative retelling of the trauma story, and (3) restoring the connection between survivors and their community" (p. 3). In addition, this approach follows neuro-physiological recommendations to begin with lower brain regions to establish a sense of safety and self-regulation (lower brain mediated) before progressing to insightful reflection, trauma experience integration, relational engagement, or positive affect enhancement (higher brain mediated) (Gaskill and Perry, 2012).

For groups of children who are experiencing bereavement and loss, TICCPT sessions are divided into four parts: (a) 5-minute opening ice breaker activity and check-in; (b) 25 minutes of CCPT; (c) 25 minutes of psycho-education activities (e.g., Theraplay® and TF-CBT); and (d) 5 minutes of calm closure. The grief group meets for 10 group 1-hour sessions and two individual 1-hour sessions for each child. The 10 group session objectives, ice breaker activities, and psycho-educational activities that facilitate children's achievement of Baker et al.'s (1992) tasks for uncomplicated grief are listed in Table 14.1.

Opening

Beginning each session with an opening ice-breaker activity and check-in provides a predictable ritual in a disrupted world for grieving children. For the first session, the play therapist leads children in a nonthreatening ice-breaker activity such as the name game (described in Chapter 12 and Table 14.1). Then, children are instructed to sit on the floor in a circle. The play therapist says "Thank you for coming to our group today. This group is for children like you who had someone special die or leave. The purpose of our group is to provide a safe and fun place for you to play and learn. Each week, we are going to spend 5 minutes doing an ice-breaker activity and checking-in with each other. Then you get to play for 25 minutes. After that we will have a snack while we do an activity for 25 minutes and then wrap up with a 5 minute calm closing activity." During this first session introduction, the play therapist also reviews confidentiality. In subsequent sessions, the play therapist begins with the ice-breaker activity listed in Table 14.1. Then the play therapist conducts the check-in by passing a colorful "talking stick." When holding the talking stick, the child identifies one positive occurrence during the week and expresses one negative occurrence or concern.

Table 14.1   Activities for Grief Group

Session objective	Ice-breaker	Psycho-education activity
Demonstrate physiological self-regulation skills.	Review group purpose, confidentiality, and safety. Name Game: Child says "I am ___" in a silly voice followed by others saying "You are ___" in the same silly voice three times. (Theraplay®)	Sensory motor activities of rocking, dance, and finger painting. Gross motor activities of yoga and Theraplay® activities.
Identify coping strategies in five areas as a sense of protection of self and family from overwhelming grief and symptoms.	Bean bag toss: Stand in circle, call someone's name, and toss bean bag to them. Child catching bean bag has to name one strategy they do to calm self. Repeat five times to identify strategies for body, emotions, thoughts, behavior, and spiritual areas.	Discuss and demonstrate coping strategies to regulate five areas of body, emotions, thoughts, behavior, and spiritual. Arts and crafts activity of "Coping Heart" (see Chapter 12).
Understand the fact that someone has died and the implications of this fact.	Share, Breathe, and Clap: Sit in circle, child completes the sentence "I don't like it when someone dies because …". All participants take deep breath and clap three times while saying "yes, that stinks."	Bibliotherapy: Read book such as *I Miss You: A First Look at Death* (Thomas, 2001) and/or *When Dinosaurs Die: A Guide to Understanding Death* (Brown & Brown, 1996).

Schedule first individual session for each child to facilitate restorative trauma narrative regarding deceased person.

Accept and emotionally acknowledge the reality (and permanency) of the loss.	Picture Share:. Prior to the session, each child is asked to bring a picture of their loved one that died or was lost. Group sits in circle for each child to show picture and say "This is ___ and I really miss him/her because …" Participants listen respectfully.	Color My Feelings: Children draw an outline of their body and use different colors to represent feelings that they feel in different parts of their body (e.g., black for sadness in the heart, red for anger in hands, or green for confusion in the mind).
		Play "Garbage or Treasure" in which play therapist gives 3″ × 5″ cards with common correct and incorrect beliefs regarding death. For example, "the death was my entire fault" or "it is O.K. to be sad and cry" or "they will come back as a ghost." Then children sort out if the belief is garbage (false) or treasure (true).

Schedule second individual session for each child to facilitate restorative trauma narrative regarding deceased person.

Explore and reevaluate the relationship to the lost loved one.	Characteristic charades. Children act out one positive characteristic or memory they have of their loved one who died or was lost.	Drawing of family before and after loved one died. "In my heart forever" drawing. "Treasure box" activity.
Verbalize restorative narrative that demonstrates internalization of lost relationship with the deceased person and balanced memory of positive and negative of person that will be there for him/her over time.	Participants apply hand lotion on each other. Then they stand in circle and massage neck or upper back of other members.	"My Story Book." Participants draw pictures and/or complete sentences for their book. "Goodbye letter." Child writes or draws a goodbye letter to their deceased loved one.
Identify strategies to invest in a new relationship with others.	Balloon volley ball. Stand in circle hitting balloon in the air. When each child hits the balloon, they name one person that is kind and loving toward them.	Each child puts on a puppet show or role plays how to respond when someone asks about their deceased loved one. Children also role play how to meet new friends.
Identify strategies to return to their current developmental level and activities.	Show and Tell. Participants bring or show something that they can do or want to do well (i.e., dance, sing, play ball, etc.).	Magazine collage of what each child likes and what they would like to do. News Broadcast Talk Show Radio to problem solve (see Chapter 12).
Identify strategies to cope with the return of painful affect at different times in their developmental transitional periods.	Bubble popping. Stand in circle, play therapist, blows bubbles and names a time when children may have difficulty (i.e., anniversary of death, birthday, holiday, school play, etc.). Before children pop the bubble, they name one thing they can do to feel better.	"Car Car" Obstacle Course. Children make an obstacle course using materials in the room. One child stands behind another and puts hands on shoulder. The child in the front closes their eyes. The one behind "drives" and guides the other child through the obstacle course. Each time a barrier is reached, the child in front has to demonstrate one positive coping strategy to get through it.
Verbally share positive memories of deceased while maintaining self-regulation.	Stand in a circle. Sing "If you are healing and you know it clap your hands" to the tune of "If you are happy and you know it." Play therapist points to a child who says how they know they are healing. Continue around circle until all have spoken.	Thank you party. Children host party to say "thank you" to their caregivers. Each child shares what they have learned in the group, one positive memory they have about their deceased loved one, and one thing they are looking forward to in their future.

Child-Centered Group Play Therapy

After the 5-minute opening check-in, the play therapist initiates the 25 minutes of Child-Centered Group Play Therapy with "now, we will have our play time for 25 minutes. You can play with all the toys in most of the ways you would like." The play therapist provides children with a safe and inviting playroom that is considered a sanctuary of refuge and protection. Toys are displayed from three categories of real-life toys, aggressive release toys, and emotional release toys (Landreth, 2012). It is important to add bereavement-related toys such as toy ambulance, fire truck, and small caskets that can be used in the sand box.

Standard CCPT skills are implemented during this part of the session (Landreth, 2012). While providing therapeutic responses, the play therapist remains calm and fully attuned with children. In doing so, they produce "a harmonic emotional state that actually synchronizes their neural activity, heart rates, and hormonal systems" (Gaskill and Perry, 2012, p. 42). This process, when continuously repeated, allows children to synchronize their autonomic responses with the adult, thereby building the neuro-pathways for future adaptive self-regulation. The play therapist pays particular attention to reflect feelings of sadness, hopelessness, fear, anger, guilt, powerlessness, or joy. The play therapist also gives time and space for children to help each other. For example, Le Vieux (1999) recounted a powerful expression of grief in group play therapy.

> "It's OK to be sad and cry," said Sarah as she gently stroked Timmy's head. He looked up at her as he was burying the dad doll in the sand, "I don't like to cry because it hurts," Timmy replied. From across the room, Tom said: "Well, I sure cried a lot and then I felt good." The look on Timmy's face was one of relief as the tears welled in his eyes. Suddenly the four other children simply sat down beside him.

This interaction revealed the power of children knowing how to help each other with sadness.

While children are playing, the play therapist identifies common play themes of grieving children including searching for lost things, burying items in the sand, protecting and rescuing toys or other children from danger, moving furniture and people to new places, and good overcoming bad (Holmberg, Benedict, & Hynan, 1998; Le Vieux, 1999). Sometimes children's play themes conflict. If so, the play therapist needs to reflect feelings and facilitate understanding of children's intentions.

SUSANNA: [5-year-old Susanna spent several minutes methodically burying a toy soldier which seemed to represent her father who was killed in combat.]

PLAY THERAPIST: Susanna, you are quietly burying that one. It is important to you to make sure it is all covered up.

THOMAS: [6-year-old Thomas who witnessed his brother's drowning, runs over to the sand box.] I'll save him. [Digs up the toy soldier.]

SUSANNA: Stop it!!! [Begins to cry with eyebrows lifted and eyes wide.]

PLAY THERAPIST: Thomas, you wanted to rescue it, but Susanna, you didn't like that and maybe it even scared you.

SUSANNA: Yeah, give it back!

PLAY THERAPIST: Susanna, you are telling him that is very important to you right now and you want it back.

THOMAS: Fine, here, have it. I'll go play with something else.

SUSANNA: [Grabs the toy and begins pouring sand over it.]

PLAY THERAPIST: Thomas, you didn't know it would upset her and you decided to respect her need. You are learning to be sensitive to others. Susanna, you are learning to ask for what you need and learning to calm yourself down by pouring the sand.

In this example, the play therapist balanced children's competing needs by reflecting their feelings and intents as well as encouraging their pro-social behavior.

Psycho-Education Activities

Psycho-educational activities are implemented according to Herman's (1992) stages of establishing safety, restorative retelling of the trauma story, and connecting with supportive people. The objectives of these activities are to meet Baker et al.'s (1992) tasks for uncomplicated grief (see Table 14.1).

Establishing safety. In addition to establishing safety through a warm and inviting playroom and limit-setting, the play therapist helps children develop internal safety by teaching them physiological regulation and coping skills. Children's perception of safety is also established by explaining death and normalizing the grief process, which can decrease unspoken fears.

Physiological regulation and coping skills. In group session one, the play therapist leads children in psycho-educational activities to teach physiological regulation of their bodies (i.e., heart rate and breathing). These skills help children establish a sense of safety when they become emotionally overwhelmed. Gaskill and Perry (2012) recommended implementing neuro-sequential interventions that begin in the lower brain regions. "Using the bottom up analogy of brain processing, establishing a sense of safety and self-regulation (lower brain mediated) must supersede insightful reflection, trauma experience integration, relational engagement, or positive affect enhancement as these last elements of treatment are mediated through cortical and limbic areas (Cook et al., 2005)" (Gaskill & Perry, 2012, p. 40).

To facilitate reorganization of the brainstem, the play therapist begins with sensory motor physical sensations and preprogrammed physical action patterns. The play therapist teaches children methods to comfort themselves through replicating rhythmic sequential patterns at the heart rate of 60 beats per minute (e.g., rocking, repetitive movements of dance, singing to soft music, and drumming) (Perry, 2009; van der Kolk, 2001). Other sensory motor activities to induce a calming state include finger painting, working with clay, and playing in the sand. To facilitate reorganization of the diencephalon, the play therapist leads children through gross motor activities such as throwing balls, hula hoops, hand clapping, hop scotch, yoga, and tai chi. Other helpful activities in physiological regulation include Theraplay® activities of structure (e.g., ball throw to members with compliment), engagement (following clapping patterns), nurture (putting hand lotion on another person), and challenge (balloon volley) (Booth & Jernberg, 2010).

During group session two, children learn coping skills to regulate their body, emotions, thoughts, behavior, and spirituality. These coping skills help children develop a sense of protection of self and family from overwhelming grief. The play therapist can discuss and demonstrate the five areas of coping that are listed in Table 12.3. Each child is encouraged to commit to implement one or two activities in each of the five areas. Then children illustrate their self-selected strategies via arts and crafts activity such as "A Coping Heart" (described in Chapter 12).

Explain death and normalize the grief process.   In group session three, the play therapist explains death and normalizes the grief process by providing information. This information can decrease unspoken fear and anxiety and increase a sense of safety for children. Haine (2008) stated that children grieving a parent's death need the following information:

> (a) children whose parent has died feel a wide range of emotions, including anger and guilt; (b) the death is never the child's fault; (c) it is acceptable to talk about the parent who has died; (d) it is not unusual for children to think that they see their parent who has died or to dream about the deceased parent; and (e) children will never forget their deceased parent.
>
> (Haine, 2008, p. 114)

This information can be communicated through bibliotherapy with children's books such as *I Miss You: A First Look at Death* (Thomas, 2001) and *When Dinosaurs Die: A Guide to Understanding Death* (Brown & Brown, 1996).

Restorative retelling of trauma narrative.   A restorative retelling of a trauma narrative is necessary for children to achieve an emotional understanding and integrate the trauma as a meaningful part of their life experience (Terr, 1990; van der Kolk, 2007). A restorative retelling of a trauma narrative entails being physiologically regulated, emotionally present, and mindfully aware when explaining details about what happened and the personal meaning of the event (Cohen et al., 2006).

Individual sessions.   In order to prevent other children from being traumatized by an unprocessed narrative, it is prudent to have two individual play therapy sessions with each child (Salloum et al., 2009). During both individual sessions, the play therapist guides children to use the toys, puppets, or sandtray miniatures to (a) illustrate their relationship with the deceased person or pet prior to the death; (b) explain how and or where the person or pet died; and (c) experiences the child had after the death (i.e., attending the funeral, moving to a new home, crying, etc.). The play therapist asks the child (a) what the worst part was for the child; (b) what they wish would happen now; (c) what does this mean about the person who died, the child, and the future; and (d) what good things the deceased person or pet would want for the child (Salloum et al., 2009). During the process, the play therapist reflects feelings and content, facilitates accurate understanding, and guides the child to a restorative understanding and meaning. As needed, the play therapist helps the child to re-regulate (i.e., calm down) by allowing breaks to play or by prompting use of physiological coping skills. In other words, this is not a rigid process but rather an encouraging process. If the child does not seem ready to continue, then the play therapist allows the child to play as a method of self regulating.

Emotional and cognitive processing. In group session four, the play therapist helps children accept and emotionally acknowledge the reality and permanency of the loss. Emotions are processed by children (a) sharing photos of their loved one that died or was lost and (b) completing the color my feelings activity (O'Connor, 1983). As children share their pictures, the play therapist reflects feelings and links group members by asking who else has felt that before. Cognitive processing occurs by playing "garbage or treasure" to sort common misunderstandings (i.e., cognitive distortions) from facts about death (Felix et al., 2006). The play therapist provides accurate information as needed and prompts children to elaborate on evidence that supports the fact.

In session five, the play therapists helps children explore and reevaluate the relationship to the deceased loved one via two activities. First, play therapists ask children to draw a picture of their family doing something with the deceased loved one before he or she died. Then they are to draw a picture of their family without the deceased loved one. As each child shares their picture, the play therapist reflects feelings and thoughts. Then the play therapist guides children in the "In my heart forever" drawing. Children draw a heart on a piece of paper that represents their heart. In the heart, they draw a picture representing memories, experiences, characteristics, etc. that their loved one bestowed on them. Alternatively, the play therapist guides children in making a treasure box by decorating an old shoe box where they can keep items (e.g., pictures, drawings of memories, shells, rocks, greeting cards) that remind them of their deceased loved one (Le Vieux, 1999).

In session six, the play therapist builds on the work accomplished in the individual session by helping children verbalize a restorative retelling of the trauma narrative that demonstrates internalization of the lost relationship. This objective is accomplished by leading children in drawing and completing sentences for their individual personalized story book. Each child is given six sheets of paper that are stapled together. On the first page, they write "My story of grief by ___ [their name]." On the second page, children draw a picture of self with their loved one before he or she died. They complete the sentences "This is me and ___". "He/she was special to me because…." "Some of the fun things we used to do together were …." On the third page, children complete the sentence "On ___ [date], ___ [name of deceased] died." "Some of my feelings are …." "Some of my thoughts are …" "I will miss ___ because …" Children draw representative pictures. On the fourth page, children complete the sentence "The things I can do to feel better are ..." Children draw coping strategies. On the fifth page, children complete the sentence "the things ___ gave me that I will treasure in my heart are ..." Children draw a heart and symbols representing treasured experiences, characteristics, sayings, etc. On the sixth page, children complete the sentence "Although I feel sad and will miss ___, one positive thing I will remember is ..." Children draw a rainbow. Children are not forced to complete the activity. Rather, they are given the freedom to stop and wait quietly for others to finish. Those children who want to share their book with others are allowed to do so. The play therapist and other children affirm and encourage those children who do verbalize their restorative narrative.

The play therapist also guides children in writing or drawing a "goodbye letter" to the deceased loved one. Children are encouraged to say what they wish they could have said to the deceased loved one. Children are given an option of what to do with the letter such as put it in their treasure box, release it in a balloon, place it in a bottle, or leave it with the play therapist.

Connection with community.   Connecting with supportive and caring people helps children experience a sense of belonging in the world, which may have been lost when their loved one died. Peers are an important source of support for children. Yet, many grieving children are guarded due to feelings of awkwardness and embarrassment in responding to questions about their loved one's death. In group session seven, the play therapist helps children identify strategies to invest in new relationships with others via puppet shows and/or role playing. The play therapist demonstrates how to respond to people's questions and when to broach the topic when they need support. Then they ask children to demonstrate how to respond to different scenarios such as "what happened to your brother?" and "you seem sad today, why?" The play therapist also role plays how to meet new friends so children can experience new relationships.

In group session eight, children are encouraged to return to age-appropriate routines and activities. To accomplish this, the play therapist helps children identify their strengths and desires by having them create a magazine collage. Then, the play therapist leads children in problem solving by having them play "News Broadcast Talk Show Radio" in which children pretend to be experts who solve problems for other children (Kaduson & Schaefer, 2001). For example, after a loved one's death, some children may have started sleeping with a parent or wetting the bed again. The play therapist pretends to be a child calling into the radio show and asks the children in the group how to solve the problem. The play therapist also acts as a co-host who gives helpful information as needed.

In the ninth session, children learn to identify strategies to cope with future pain and sadness. This task allows for a helpful review of coping skills learned in sessions one and two. The play therapist and children identify vulnerable times that pain may arise such as birthdays, anniversary of death, holidays, graduation, etc. Each situation is written on a separate card. Children make an obstacle course with barriers in the room and tape cards on the barriers. Then children play "car car" obstacle course (Theraplay®, 2006). One child stands behind another and puts hands on his or her shoulders. The child in the front closes their eyes. The one behind "drives" and guides the other child through the obstacle course. Each time a barrier is reached, the child in front has to demonstrate one positive coping strategy to get through the barrier.

In the tenth group session, children demonstrate sharing positive memories of their deceased loved one while maintaining self-regulation. This is accomplished by having children plan and host a party for their parent or caregivers to say "thank you" for the support. During the party, each child thanks their caregiver and shares (a) one thing they have learned from the group; (b) a positive memory of the deceased loved one; and (c) one thing they are looking forward to in the future. Caregivers are encouraged to affirm and compliment the children on improvements they have noticed.

Calm closure.   At the end of each group session, the play therapist leads children in a 5-minute calm closing activity. This ritual helps children to re-regulate their bodies, emotions, and minds so that they can return to family members and activities in a balanced manner. To begin the calm closing activity, the play therapist asks children to sit in a circle. They listen to some meditation music, take deep breaths, and think of a calm, safe place. Short videos that serve this purpose are available online.

Conclusion

Every year, millions of U.S. children experience bereavement due to the death or loss of a significant person or pet. Bereaved children may experience physiological, cognitive, affective, behavioral, and spiritual symptoms. They may even maintain a relationship with the deceased in a fantasized way. Variables influencing children's grief responses include developmental level as well as risk and resiliency factors. Children may experience uncomplicated grief or complicated grief.

Play therapists can prepare to help bereaved children by engaging in self-reflection on their own experiences and view of death. Play therapists must carefully select compatible group members after a caregiver interview and assessment of children.

Trauma-Informed Child-Centered Group Therapy is an evidence informed approach that integrates CCPT (Landreth, 2012) with neuro-developmental activities and cognitive behavioral activities. When applied with grieving children, TICCPT sessions are formatted into: (a) 5-minute opening ice breaker activity and check-in; (b) 25 minutes of Child Centered Play Therapy; (c) 25 minutes of psycho-education activities to help children achieve tasks for uncomplicated grief; and (d) 5 minutes of calm closure. The grief group meets for 10 group 1-hour sessions and two individual 1-hour sessions for each child.

By implementing this recommended TICCPT grief group curriculum, play therapists will help children establish safety, engage in a restorative retelling of their trauma narrative, and connect with supportive people in their community. This process will facilitate healing in bereaved children and prepare them to live with meaning in the future.

15 Research and Outcomes in Group Play Therapy

Overall, research indicates that group play therapy is an effective intervention for children who present with varied problems. In a meta-analysis of 93 play therapy studies including 33 group play studies, Bratton, Ray, Rhine, and Jones (2005) found similar outcomes between group and individual play therapy, reporting a Cohen's d effect size of .82 for group play therapy. In a meta-analysis of 42 play therapy studies, LeBlanc and Ritchie (2001) reported no significant differences between outcomes of individual and group play therapy studies, indicating that individual and group play therapy are both equally effective.

Research in group play therapy spans over 70 years and multiple topics of focus. Early studies were specifically interested in the relationship between group play therapy and intelligence (e.g., Bills, 1950a, 1950b; Cowen & Cruickshank, 1948; Cruickshank & Cowen, 1948). More recent studies have explored the impact of group play therapy on specific disorders and trauma (e.g., Jalali & Molavi, 2011; Mahmoudi-Gharaei, Bina, Yasami, Emami, & Naderi, 2006). As would be expected, several studies concentrated on the effect of group play therapy on social adjustment (e.g., Thombs & Muro, 1973; Trostle, 1988). In a review of group play therapy literature published since 1940, we identified 32 studies using group play therapy as the identified experimental condition. Table 15.1 includes a breakdown of number of studies per decade.

The publication of such a large number of studies indicates that group play therapy is an intervention of interest to the mental health field. Considering that the majority of group intervention studies involving children are short-term, nonexperimental, cognitive-behaviorally oriented, highly structured, and designed for children aged 9–12 years old (Reddy, 2012), we were surprised to locate a substantial number of studies on group play therapy. Typically, studies involving group interventions for children

Table 15.1 Group Play Therapy Research Publications Per Decade

1940	1950	1960	1970	1980	1990	2000	2010
3	5	3	9	3	0	6	3

do not utilize the modality of play to communicate with children. Of the studies identified for this chapter, research concentrated on intervention for children 4–12 years old, with the majority of studies conducted with children under 10 years old. Research conducted with this age group signifies that group play therapy is a viable intervention for young children.

Regarding theoretical approach to group play therapy, 24 of the 32 identified studies reported a nondirective approach to intervention. The nondirective label includes interventions based on child-centered play therapy (CCPT), relationship play therapy, self-directive play therapy, and psychoanalytic play therapy. As found in previous reviews of play therapy research literature (Ray, 2011), the majority of play therapy research is based on the CCPT philosophy to intervention. Research in group play therapy follows the same pattern. A few studies (n=5) explored the use of more directive approaches such as behavioral, Gestalt, cognitive-behavioral play therapy, and developmental play therapy. Two studies did not identify the type of play therapy utilized. Newcomer and Morrison (1974) specifically compared the use of nondirective, directive, group and individual play therapy and found no differences between the modalities.

In order to identify group play therapy research studies for this chapter, we used the following criteria: (1) group play therapy was clearly used as the research intervention signified by the use of the phrases "play therapy" or "play counseling" in relation to a group format; (2) study was published in a journal or dissertation; (3) play therapy was facilitated for children, not parents or families; and (4) study utilized aspects of experimental design. The restriction of criteria to the use of the phrase "play therapy" limited the inclusion of more cognitive-behavioral group interventions that use games or materials but do not identify as play therapy. Knell and Dasari (2011) cited 20 case studies of cognitive-behavioral play therapy (CBPT) discussed in published literature. However, many of the case studies are lacking assessments to measure change. Furthermore, Knell and Dasari noted the lack of randomized, clinical intervention studies in CBPT.

The remainder of this chapter includes a brief synopsis of the 32 group play therapy studies categorized by research issue (Tables 15.2–15.13). Research issues are: externalizing/disruptive behaviors (n=4), attention deficit hyperactivity disorder (n=1), internalizing behavior problems (n=4), anxiety (n=6), depression (n=2), self-concept/self-esteem (n=6), social behavior (n=10), trauma/abuse (n=4), homelessness (n=1), identified disability/medical condition (n=5), academic achievement/intelligence (n=6), and speech/language skills (n=3). Some studies are listed in multiple categories due to outcomes related to more than one area.

Table 15.2 Research Issue: Externalizing/Disruptive Behavior Problems

Author/s	# Participants— Ages	Description
Fleming & Snyder (1947)	7—Ages 8–11	Authors found that after 12 nondirective group play therapy sessions, girls' group showed significant improvement in personality adjustment as compared to control group.
Gaulden (1975)	45—2nd graders	Author found that when comparing 14 sessions of developmental play group, 14 sessions of play group counseling, and nonintervention control group, children in play therapy group scored significantly lower on classroom disturbance than other experimental groups.
Packman & Bratton (2003)	24—Ages 10–12	Authors found that after 12 humanistically oriented group play therapy sessions, preadolescents with learning disabilities and exhibiting behavioral problems showed statistically significant improvement on externalizing problems and total problems.
Tyndall-Lind, Landreth, & Giordano (2001)	32—Ages 4–10	Authors compared a sibling group play therapy condition to an intensive individual play therapy condition and a control condition for children living in a domestic violence shelter. Sibling group CCPT consisted of 12 sessions of 45 minutes over 12 days. Results indicated that sibling group play therapy was equally effective to intensive individual play therapy. Children in sibling group play therapy demonstrated a significant reduction in total behavior, externalizing, and internalizing behavior problems, aggression, anxiety, and depression and significant improvement in self-esteem.

Table 15.3 Research Issue: Attention Deficit Hyperactivity Disorder (ADHD)

Author/s	# Participants— Ages	Description
Naderi, Heidarie, Bouron, & Asgari (2010)	80—Ages 8–12	Authors found that children diagnosed with ADHD demonstrated statistically significant improvement on ADHD symptoms, anxiety, and social maturity following 10 sessions of group play therapy using mixed collection of play and games, when compared to a randomized control group.

Table 15.4 Research Issue: Internalizing Behavior Problems

Author/s	# Participants— Ages	Description
Clement, Fazzone, & Goldstein (1970)	16—2nd & 3rd grade	Authors compared boys who were shy and withdrawn under four conditions including a play group that received token reinforcement for 20 sessions. Results demonstrated that the token play group improved significantly over other groups on classroom behavior and personality adjustment.
Clement & Milne (1967)	11—3rd grade	Authors found that boys who were shy and withdrawn participating in 14 sessions of token group play therapy exhibited an increase in social approach behavior and decrease in problem behavior over boys who participated in a verbal play group or comparison control group.
Fleming & Snyder (1947)	7—Ages 8–11	Authors found that after 12 nondirective group play therapy sessions, girls' group showed significant improvement in personality adjustment as compared to control group.
Tyndall-Lind, Landreth, & Giordano (2001)	32—Ages 4–10	Authors compared a sibling group play therapy condition to an intensive individual play therapy condition and a control condition for children living in a domestic violence shelter. Sibling group CCPT consisted of 12 sessions of 45 minutes over 12 days. Results indicated that sibling group play therapy was equally effective to intensive individual play therapy. Children in sibling group play therapy demonstrated a significant reduction in total behavior, externalizing, and internalizing behavior problems, aggression, anxiety, and depression and significant improvement in self-esteem.

Table 15.5   Research Issue: Anxiety

Author/s	# Participants— Ages	Description
Baggerly (2004)	42—Ages 5–11	Author conducted a pretest posttest single group design for children living in a homeless shelter. Children participated in 9–12 group CCPT sessions of 30 minutes once or twice a week. Results revealed significant improvement in self-concept, significance, competence, negative mood and negative self-esteem related to depression, and anxiety.
Farahzadi, Bahramabadi, & Mohammadifar (2011)	12—Age 11	Authors found that children who participated in 10 sessions of Gestalt group play therapy demonstrated a reduction in social phobia symptoms as compared to children in control group.
Jalali & Molavi (2011)	30—Ages 5–11	Authors found that children who participated in six group play therapy sessions demonstrated statistically significant reduction in separation anxiety as compared to a no-treatment control group. Type of play therapy was not specified in translated abstract.
Naderi, Heidarie, Bouron, & Asgari (2010)	80—Ages 8–12	Authors found that children diagnosed with ADHD demonstrated statistically significant improvement on ADHD symptoms, anxiety, and social maturity following 10 sessions of group play therapy using mixed collection of play and games, when compared to a randomized control group.
Shen (2002)	30—Ages 8–12	Author randomly assigned child participants from a rural elementary school in Taiwan following an earthquake to a CCPT group or control group. All children were scored at high risk for maladjustment. The CCPT groups received 10 group play therapy sessions of 40 minutes, over 4 weeks. Results indicated the CCPT group demonstrated a significant decrease in anxiety, as well as a large treatment effect, and significant decrease in suicide risk as compared to the control group.
Tyndall-Lind, Landreth, & Giordano (2001)	32—Ages 4–10	Authors compared a sibling group play therapy condition to an intensive individual play therapy condition and a control condition for children living in a domestic violence shelter. Sibling group CCPT consisted of 12 sessions of 45 minutes over 12 days. Results indicated that sibling group play therapy was equally effective to intensive individual play therapy. Children in sibling group play therapy demonstrated a significant reduction in total behavior, externalizing, and internalizing behavior problems, aggression, anxiety, and depression and significant improvement in self-esteem.

Table 15.6 Research Issue: Depression

Author/s	# Participants— Ages	Description
Baggerly (2004)	42—Ages 5–11	Author conducted a pretest posttest single group design for children living in a homeless shelter. Children participated in 9–12 CCPT group play therapy sessions of 30 minutes, once or twice a week. Results revealed significant improvement in self-concept, significance, competence, negative mood and negative self-esteem related to depression, and anxiety.
Tyndall-Lind, Landreth, & Giordano (2001)	32—Ages 4–10	Authors compared a sibling group play therapy condition to an intensive individual play therapy condition and a control condition for children living in a domestic violence shelter. Sibling group CCPT consisted of 12 sessions of 45 minutes over 12 days. Results indicated that sibling group play therapy was equally effective to intensive individual play therapy. Children in sibling group play therapy demonstrated a significant reduction in total behavior, externalizing, and internalizing behavior problems, aggression, anxiety, and depression, and significant improvement in self-esteem.

Table 15.7   Research Issue: Self-Concept/Self-Esteem

Author/s	# Participants— Ages	Description
Baggerly (2004)	42—Ages 5–11	Author conducted a pretest posttest single group design for children living in a homeless shelter. Children participated in 9–12 CCPT group play therapy sessions of 30 minutes, once or twice a week. Results revealed significant improvement in self-concept, significance, competence, negative mood and negative self-esteem related to depression, and anxiety.
Gould (1980)	84—Elementary school	Author found that children identified as having a low self-image who participated in 12 sessions of nondirective group play therapy and those who participated in a placebo of 12 discussion groups showed positive improvement on self-concept as compared to no change in the nonintervention control group. The strongest positive change was noted for the group play therapy participants.
House (1970)	36—2nd graders	Author found after 20 sessions of child-centered group play therapy, socially maladjusted children significantly increased self-concept while members of the control group decreased in self-concept.
Pelham (1972)	52— kindergarteners	Author found that in comparing socially immature kindergartners participating in 6–8 individual self-directive play therapy sessions, 6–8 group self-directive play therapy sessions, or a control group, children in both treatment groups made positive gains in social maturity when compared to control group. Children participating in play therapy improved significantly in classroom behavior when compared to control group.
Perez (1987)	55—Ages 4–9	Author found that in comparing sexually abused children participating in 12 sessions of individual relationship play therapy, 12 sessions of group relationship play therapy, or a control group, self-concepts of children in treatment groups increased at a significant level while those in control group actually decreased. The self-mastery scores of children in play therapy rose significantly while those in control group dropped. No differences found between individual and group play therapy.
Tyndall-Lind, Landreth, & Giordano (2001)	32—Ages 4–10	Authors compared a sibling group play therapy condition to an intensive individual play therapy condition and a control condition for children living in a domestic violence shelter. Sibling group CCPT consisted of 12 sessions of 45 minutes over 12 days. Results indicated that sibling group play therapy was equal in effectiveness to intensive individual play therapy. Children in sibling group play therapy demonstrated a significant reduction in total behavior, externalizing, and internalizing behavior problems, aggression, anxiety, and depression and significant improvement in self-esteem.

Table 15.8 Research Issue: Social Behavior

Author/s	# Participants— Ages	Description
Elliott & Pumfrey (1972)	28—Ages 7–9	Authors found that after 9 sessions of nondirective group play therapy, boys rated no differences on social adjustment or reading attainment than a control group receiving no intervention. However, interaction was demonstrated between improvement and selection criteria such as IQ; emotional disturbance, which improved on social adjustment with therapy; and restlessness, which deteriorated in social adjustment with therapy.
Fleming & Snyder (1947)	46—Ages 8–11	Authors found that after 12 nondirective group play therapy sessions, girls' group showed significant improvement in personality adjustment as compared to control group.
House (1970)	36—2nd graders	Author found after 20 sessions of child-centered group play therapy, socially maladjusted children significantly increased self-concept while members of the control group decreased in self-concept.
Hume (1967)	20—1st—4th graders	Author found that after 6 months of weekly child-centered individual and group play therapy sessions with or without teacher inservice focusing on creating growth conditions in the classroom, play therapy participants showed considerable improvement in their behavior in school, at home and in play therapy by end of school year and at follow-up. Play therapy appeared to be most effective when combined with teacher in-service, yet in-service appeared to be only partially helpful without play therapy.
Naderi, Heidarie, Bouron, & Asgari (2010)	80—Ages 8–12	Authors found that children diagnosed with ADHD demonstrated statistically significant improvement on ADHD symptoms, anxiety, and social maturity following 10 sessions of group play therapy using mixed collection of play and games, when compared to a randomized control group.
Pelham (1972)	52—kindergarteners	Author found that in comparing socially immature kindergartners participating in 6–8 individual self-directive play therapy sessions, 6–8 group self-directive play therapy sessions, or a control group, children in both treatment groups made positive gains in social maturity when compared to control group. Children participating in play therapy improved significantly in classroom behavior when compared to control group.
Schiffer (1966)	33—Ages 9–11	Author found that after 6½ months of weekly sessions comparing group play therapy with parents, group play therapy without parents, recreation group, and control group, children in the treatment groups stabilized in peer relationships while control group children increased in social maladjustment.

(*continued*)

Table 15.8   Continued

Author/s	# Participants— Ages	Description
Sokoloff (1959)	24—Age 5	Author found that when comparing 30 sessions of group play therapy to 30 sessions of individual speech therapy for children with cerebral palsy, children who participated in play therapy improved in speech and communication, as well as social development.
Thombs & Muro (1973)	36—2nd graders	Authors found that after 15 sessions of relationship theory-based group play therapy, children showed a greater positive change in social position than those who participated in the alternate verbal group counseling experimental group. Both experimental groups made significant gains in sociometric status as compared to control group.
Trostle (1988)	48—Ages 3–6	Authors found that after 10 sessions of nondirective group play therapy, bilingual Puerto Rican children showed significant improvement compared to control group on self-control, and the higher developmental level play behaviors of make-believe and reality. Boys who participated in the experimental group became more accepting of others than boys or girls in the control group. The control group participated in unstructured free play sessions as opposed to group play therapy sessions.

Table 15.9   Research Issue: Trauma/Abuse

Author/s	# Participants— Ages	Description
Mahmoudi-Gharaei, Bina, Yasami, Emami, & Naderi (2006)	13—Ages 3–6	Authors found that children who had experienced an earthquake in which they lost a family member demonstrated a statistically significant reduction in trauma-related symptoms after participating in 12 cognitive-behavioral group play therapy sessions.
Perez (1987)	55—Ages 4–9	Author found that in comparing sexually abused children participating in 12 sessions of individual relationship play therapy, 12 sessions of group relationship play therapy, or a control group, self-concepts of children in treatment groups increased at a significant level, while those in control group actually decreased. The self-mastery scores of children in play therapy rose significantly, while those in control group dropped. No differences found between individual and group play therapy.
Shen (2002)	30—Ages 8–12	Author randomly assigned child participants from a rural elementary school in Taiwan to a CCPT group or control group following an earthquake. All children were scored at high risk for maladjustment. The CCPT groups received 10 group play therapy sessions of 40 minutes over 4 weeks. Results indicated the CCPT group demonstrated a significant decrease in anxiety, as well as a large treatment effect, and significant decrease in suicide risk as compared to the control group.
Tyndall-Lind, Landreth, & Giordano (2001)	32—Ages 4–10	Authors compared a sibling group play therapy condition to an intensive individual play therapy condition and a control condition for children living in a domestic violence shelter. Sibling group CCPT consisted of 12 sessions of 45 minutes over 12 days. Results indicated that sibling group play therapy was equal in effectiveness to intensive individual play therapy. Children in sibling group play therapy demonstrated a significant reduction in total behavior, externalizing, and internalizing behavior problems, aggression, anxiety, and depression and significant improvement in self-esteem.

Table 15.10   Research Issue: Homelessness

Author/s	# Participants— Ages	Description
Baggerly (2004)	42—Ages 5-11	Author conducted a pretest posttest single group design for children living in a homeless shelter. Children participated in 9–12 CCPT group play therapy sessions of 30 minutes, once or twice a week. Results revealed significant improvement in self-concept, significance, competence, negative mood and negative self-esteem related to depression, and anxiety.

Table 15.11   Research Issue: Identified Disability/Medical Condition

Author/s	# Participants— Ages	Description
Cruickshank & Cowen (1948) and Cowen & Cruickshank (1948)	5—Ages 7–9	Authors found that of five physically handicapped children identified as having emotional problems in school who received 13 nondirective group play therapy sessions, three children showed considerable improvement in behavior at home and at school, one showed some slight evidences of gain, while the fifth gave no indication of any improvement. All five reported positive feelings toward experience.
Danger & Landreth (2005)	21—Ages 4–6	Authors randomly assigned children qualified for speech therapy to one of two conditions including group play therapy condition and regularly scheduled speech therapy session condition. Children assigned to the play therapy condition received 25 sessions of group CCPT concurrently with speech therapy over 7 months. Results revealed that children in play therapy demonstrated increased receptive language skills and expressive language skills with large practical significance.
Mehlman (1953)	32—Ages 86–140 months	Author found that when comparing 29 sessions of group play therapy, movie group, and nonintervention group, children with intellectual disabilities showed no changes in intelligence among any group. The play therapy group showed improvement on personality adjustment.
Sokoloff (1959)	24—Age 5	Author found that when comparing 30 sessions of group play therapy to 30 sessions of individual speech therapy for children with cerebral palsy, children who participated in play therapy improved in speech and communication, as well as social development.

Table 15.12   Research Issue: Academic Achievement/Intelligence

Author/s	# Participants— Ages	Description
Bills (1950a)	18—3rd graders	Author found that emotionally maladjusted children receiving 6 individual child-centered play therapy sessions and 3 group play therapy sessions showed significant improvement on reading ability and maintained improvement 30 days after intervention as compared to a control group.
Bills (1950b)	8—3rd graders	Author also found that well-adjusted children who received nondirective individual and group play therapy failed to make statistically significant gains in reading ability following nondirective play therapy. He concluded from these two studies that reading gains noted in maladjusted slow readers followed a nondirective treatment of the maladjustment present in the children.
Elliott & Pumfrey (1972)	28—Ages 7–9	Authors found that after 9 sessions of nondirective group play therapy, boys rated no differences on social adjustment or reading attainment than a control group receiving no intervention. However, interaction was demonstrated between improvement and selection criteria such as IQ; emotional disturbance, which improved on social adjustment with therapy; and restlessness, which deteriorated in social adjustment with therapy.
Mehlman (1953)	32—Ages 86–140 months	Author found that when comparing 29 sessions of group play therapy, movie group, and nonintervention group, children with intellectual disabilities showed no changes in intelligence among any group. The play therapy group showed improvement on personality adjustment.
Newcomer & Morrison (1974)	12—Ages 5–11	Authors found that when comparing individual play therapy with directive and nondirective leadership to group play therapy with directive and nondirective leadership, the mean scores of both treatment groups comprised of children with intellectual disabilities increased continuously over 30 weeks. A beneficial effect on social and intellectual functioning was shown as compared to the control group. There were no differences between group versus individual or directive versus nondirective.
Seeman & Edwards (1954)	38—5th—6th graders	Authors found that personally maladjusted children who received an average of 67 sessions of play groups led by a "teacher-therapist" maintaining a child-centered atmosphere made a significant reading gain of 7/10 of a year in 4 months in comparison to a control group.

Table 15.13   Research Issue: Speech/Language Skills

Author/s	# Participants— Ages	Description
Bouillion (1974)	43—Ages 3–6	Author compared children with a speech or language delay through treatment groups of nondirective group play therapy, individual direct speech therapy, group speech lessons, and physical-motor training that met 5 days a week for 14 weeks with a nonintervention control group. Children who participated in group play therapy achieved significantly higher scores than the other treatment groups in the areas of fluency and articulation. Play therapy group also showed the least improvement in remediating receptive language deficits.
Danger & Landreth (2005)	21—Ages 4–6	Authors randomly assigned children qualified for speech therapy to one of two conditions including group play therapy condition and regularly scheduled speech therapy session condition. Children assigned to the play therapy condition received 25 sessions of group CCPT concurrently with speech therapy over 7 months. Results revealed that children in play therapy demonstrated increased receptive language skills and expressive language skills with large practical significance.
Moulin (1970)	126—1st–3rd graders	Author found after 12 sessions of client-centered group play therapy, underachieving students made significantly greater gains in non-language intelligence than the control group. Treatment was effective in significantly increasing meaningful language usage, not automatic language. There was no effect on academic achievement.

References

Abramson, D., Stehling-Ariza, T., Garfield, R., & Redlener, I. (2008). Prevalence and predictors of mental health distress post-Katrina: Findings from the Gulf Coast Child and Family Health Study. *Disaster Medicine and Public Health Preparedness, 2*(2), 77–86.

Allan, J. (1988). *Inscapes of the child's world: Jungian counseling in schools and clinics.* Dallas, TX: Spring.

Allan, J. (1997). Jungian play psychotherapy. In K. O'Connor & L. Braverman (Eds.), *Play therapy: A comparative presentation* (2nd ed., pp. 100–130). New York: Wiley.

Allan, J., & Bertoia, J. (2003). *Written paths to healing: Education and Jungian child counseling.* Putnam, CT: Spring.

American Art Therapy Association (2012). *Art therapy: Definition of the profession.* Available at http://arttherapy.org/aata-aboutus.html

American Psychological Association (2000). *Diagnostic and statistical manual of mental disorders. DSM-IV-TR* (4th ed.: text revision). Washington, DC: Author.

American Psychological Association Presidential Task Force on Evidence Based Practice (2006). Evidence-based practice in psychology. *American Psychologist, 61,* 271–285.

Andrews, C. (2009). *Who directs the play and why? An exploratory study of directive versus non-directive play therapy.* Master's Thesis, Smith College for Social Work, Northampton, MA.

Arnett, J.J. (1999). Adolescent storm and stress, reconsidered. *American Psychologist, 54*(5), 317–326.

Ashby, J., Kottman, T., & DeGraaf, D. (2008). *Active interventions for kids and teens: Adding adventures and fun to counseling.* Alexandria, VA: American Counseling Association.

Association for Play Therapy. (2009). *Play therapy best practices.* Fresno, CA: Association for Play Therapy.

Association for Specialists in Group Work. (2000). *Professional standards for the training of group workers.* Alexandria, VA: Association for Specialists in Group Work.

Atkins, S. (2002). *Expressive arts therapy: Creative process in art and life.* Boone, NC: Parkway.

Axford, N., & Morpeth, L. (2013). Evidence-based programs in children's services: A critical appraisal. *Children and Youth Services Review, 35,* 266–277.

Axline, V. (1947). *Play therapy.* New York: Ballantine.

Axline, V. (1949). Mental deficiency: Symptom or disease? *Journal of Consulting Psychology, 13,* 313–327.

Baggerly, J. (2004). The effects of child-centered group play therapy on self-concept, depression, and anxiety on children who are homeless. *International Journal of Play Therapy, 13,* 31–51.

Baggerly, J.N. (2006a). *Disaster mental health and crisis stabilization for children* (Video). Framingham, MA: Microtraining Associates.

Baggerly, J.N. (2006b). Preparing play therapists for disaster response: Principles and procedures. *International Journal of Play Therapy, 15,* 59–82.

Baggerly, J.N. (2007). International interventions and challenges following the crisis of natural disasters. In N.B. Webb (Ed.), *Play therapy with children in crisis* (3 ed., pp. 345–367). New York: Guilford Press.

Baggerly, J.N. (2010). Systematic trauma interventions for children: A 10 step protocol. In J. Webber (Ed.), *Terrorism, trauma, and tragedies: A counselor's guide to preparing and responding* (2nd ed., pp. 131–136). Alexandria, VA: American Counseling Association.

Baggerly, J. (2012). *Trauma-informed child-centered play therapy* (Video). Framingham, MA: Microtraining Associates and Alexander Street Press.

Baggerly, J.N., & Exum, H. (2008). Counseling children after natural disasters: Guidance for family therapists. *American Journal of Family Therapy, 36*(1), 79–93.

Baggerly, J., & Ferretti, L. (2008). The impact of the 2004 hurricanes on Florida comprehensive assessment test scores: Implications for school counselors. *Professional School Counseling, 12,* 1–9.

Baggerly, J.N., & Mescia, N. (2005). *Disaster behavioral health first aid specialist training with children: C-FAST.* Tampa, FL: Florida Center for Public Health Preparedness.

Baggerly, J., & Parker, M. (2005). Child-centered group play therapy with African American boys at the elementary school level. *Journal of Counseling & Development, 83*(4), 387–396.

Baggerly, J., Green, C., Thorn, A., & Steele, W. (2007). He blew our house down: Natural disaster and trauma. In S. Dugger & L. Carlson (Eds.), *Critical Incidents in Counseling Children* (pp. 71–80). Alexandria, VA: American Counseling Association Press.

Baggerly, J., Ray, D., & Bratton, S. (Eds.) (2010). *Child-centered play therapy research: The evidence base for effective practice.* Hoboken, NJ: John Wiley.

Baker, J., Sedney, M., & Gross, E. (1992). Psychological tasks for bereaved children. *American Journal of Orthopsychiatry, 62*(1), 105–116.

Baker, S.R. (2005). *Freedom and death.* Tampa, FL: The Life Center of the Suncoast Inc.

Bandura, A. (1977). *Social learning theory.* Oxford: Prentice-Hall.

Barbarin, O.A. (1993). Emotional and social development of African American children. *Journal of Black Psychology, 19*(4), 381–390.

Beck, A. (1976). *Cognitive therapy and the emotional disorders.* New York: Meridian.

Beck, A., & Weishaar, M. (2005). Cognitive therapy. In R. Corsini & D. Wedding (Eds.), *Current psychotherapies* (7th ed., pp. 238–268). Belmont, CA: Thomson.

Beck, A., & Weishaar, M. (2008). Cognitive therapy. In R. Corsini & D. Wedding (Eds.), *Current psychotherapies* (8th ed., pp. 263–294). Belmont, CA: Thomson.

Beck, J.S. (2011). *Cognitive behavior therapy: Basics and beyond* (2nd ed.). New York: Guilford Press.

Becker-Blease, K.A., Turner, H.A., & Finkelhor, D. (2010). Disasters, victimization, and children's mental health. *Child Development, 81,* 1040–1052.

Berg, R.C., Landreth, G.L., & Fall, K.A. (2006). *Group counseling: Concepts and procedures* (3rd ed.). New York: Routledge/Taylor & Francis.

Bergin, J., & Klein, J. (2009). Small-group counseling. In A. Vernon (Ed.), *Counseling children and adolescents* (4th ed., pp. 359–386). Denver, CO: Love.

Berk, L.E. (2010). *Exploring lifespan development* (2nd ed.). Boston, MA: Allyn & Bacon.

Bertoia, J. (1999). The invisible village: Jungian group play therapy. In D. Sweeney & L. Homeyer (Eds.), *The handbook of group play therapy: How to do it, how it works, whom it's best for* (pp. 86–104). San Francisco, CA: Jossey-Bass.

Bills, R. (1950a). Nondirective play therapy with retarded readers. *Journal of Consulting Psychology, 14,* 140–149.

Bills, R. (1950b). Play therapy with well-adjusted retarded readers. *Journal of Consulting Psychology, 14*, 246–249.

Bishop, C.M. (2011). How visible and integrated are lesbian, gay, bisexual, and transgender families: A survey of school psychologists regarding school characteristics. *Dissertation Abstracts International, 72*.

Blanco, P., & Ray, D. (2011). Play therapy in the schools: A best practice for improving academic achievement. *Journal of Counseling and Development, 89*, 235–242.

Blanco, P., Ray, D., & Holliman, R. (2012). Long-term child centered play therapy and academic achievement of children: A follow-up study. *International Journal of Play Therapy, 21*, 1–13.

Blom, R. (2006). *The handbook of gestalt play therapy: Practical guidelines for child therapists.* London: Jessica Kingsley.

Blundon, J., & Schaefer, C. (2006). The use of group play therapy for children with social skills deficits. In H. Kaduson & C. Schaefer (Eds.), *Short-term play therapy for children* (2nd ed., pp. 336–375). New York: Guilford.

Booth, P., & Jernberg, A. (2010). *Theraplay: Helping parents and children build better relationships through attachment-based play.* San Francisco, CA: Jossey-Bass.

Bouillion, K. (1974). The comparative efficacy of non-directive group play therapy with preschool, speech- or language-delayed children (Doctoral dissertation, Texas Tech University, 1973). *Dissertation Abstracts International, 35*, 495.

Bozarth, J. (1998). *Person-centered therapy: A revolutionary paradigm.* Ross-on-Wye: PCCS Books.

Brabender, V. (2002). *Introduction to group therapy.* New York: John Wiley & Sons.

Bratton, S., & Ferebee, K. (1999). The use of structured expressive art activities in group activity therapy with preadolescents. In D.S. Sweeney & L.E. Homeyer (Eds.), *The handbook of group play therapy: How to do it, how it works, whom it's best for* (pp. 192–214). San Francisco, CA: Jossey-Bass.

Bratton, S., & Ray, D. (1999). Group puppetry. In D. Sweeney & L. Homeyer (Eds.), *The handbook of group play therapy: How to do it, how it works, whom it's best for* (pp. 267–277). San Francisco, CA: Jossey-Bass.

Bratton, S., Ray, D., Rhine, T., & Jones, L. (2005). The efficacy of play therapy with children: A meta-analytic review. *Professional Psychology: Research and Practice, 36*, 376–390.

Briere, J. (1996). *Trauma symptom checklist for children.* Odessa, FL: Psychological Assessment Resources.

Briere, J. (2005). *Trauma Symptom Checklist for Young Children (TSCYC): Professional Manual.* Odessa, FL: Psychological Assessment Resources.

Briggs, K., Runyon, M., & Deblinger, E. (2011). The use of play in trauma-focused cognitive-behavioral therapy. In S. Russ & L. Niec (Eds.), *Play in clinical practice: Evidence-based approaches* (pp. 168–200). New York: Guilford.

Bromfield, R. (1995). The use of puppets in play therapy. *Child and Adolescent Social Work Journal, 12*, 435–444.

Brown, K.L., & Brown, M. (1996). *When dinosaurs die: A guide to understanding death.* New York: Little, Brown Books for Young Readers.

Brymer, M., Jacobs, A., Layne, C., Pynoos, R., Ruzek, J., Steinberg, A., Vernberg, E., & Watson, P. (National Child Traumatic Stress Network and National Center for PTSD) (2006). *Psychological First Aid: Field Operations Guide* (2nd ed.) July, 2006. Retrieved from www.nctsn.org and www.ncptsd.va.gov

Bunge, S.A. (2009). *The adolescent brain.* Available from www.youtube.com/watch?v=7GSVja_AO-Q

Burns, R.C., & Kaufman, S. (1980). *Kinetic family drawings (K-F-D).* New York: Brunner/Mazel.

Butler, S., Guterman, J., & Rudes, J. (2009). Using puppets with children in narrative therapy to externalize the problem. *Journal of Mental Health Counseling, 31,* 225–233.

Carey, L. (2006). *Expressive and creative arts methods for trauma survivors.* London: Jessica Kingsley.

Carlson-Sabelli, L. (1998). Children's therapeutic puppet theatre—Action, interaction, and cocreation. *International Journal of Action Methods, 51,* 91–112.

Carroll, F. (2009). Gestalt play therapy. In K. O'Connor & L. Braverman (Eds.), *Play therapy theory and practice: Comparing theories and techniques* (2nd ed., pp. 283–314). Hoboken, NJ: Wiley.

Carter, R., & Mason, P. (1998). The selection and use of puppets in counseling. *Professional School Counseling, 1,* 50–53.

Casey, B.J., Jones, R.M., Levita, L., Libby, V., Pattwell, S.S., Ruberry, E.J., Soliman, F., & Somerville, L.H. (2010). The storm and stress of adolescence: Insights from human imaging and mouse genetics. *Developmental Psychobiology, 52,* 225–235.

Celano, M.P. (1990). Activities and games for group psychotherapy with sexually abused children. *International Journal of Group Psychotherapy, 40,* 419–429.

Center for Disease Control (2011). *National Vital Statistics Reports. Death: Final Date for 2010.* Atlanta, GA: Center for Disease Control.

Chapman, L., & Appleton, V. (1999). Art in group play therapy. In D.S. Sweeney & L.E. Homeyer (Eds.), *The handbook of group play therapy: How to do it, how it works, whom it's best for* (pp. 179–191). San Francisco, CA: Jossey-Bass.

Christner, R., Stewart, J., & Freeman, A. (2007). *Handbook of cognitive-behavior group therapy with children and adolescents: Specific settings and presenting problems.* New York: Routledge.

Clement, P., & Milne, D. (1967). Group play therapy and tangible reinforcers used to modify the behavior of 8-year-old boys. *Behaviour Research and Therapy, 5,* 301–312.

Clement, P., Fazzone, R., & Goldstein, B. (1970). Tangible reinforcers and child group therapy. *Journal of the American Academy of Child Psychiatry, 9,* 409–427.

Cobia, D., & Henderson, D. (2007). *Developing an effective and accountable school counseling program* (2nd ed.). Upper Saddle River, NJ: Pearson Education.

Cochran, N., Nordling, W., & Cochran, J. (2010). *Child-centered play therapy: A practical guide to developing therapeutic relationships with children.* Hoboken, NJ: Wiley.

Cohen, J.A., Mannarino, A.P., & Deblinger, E. (2006). *Treating trauma and traumatic grief in children and adolescents.* New York: Guilford.

Cohen, J.A., Mannarino, A.P., & Deblinger, E. (2012). *Trauma-focused CBT for children and adolescents: Treatment applications.* New York: Guilford.

Constantine, M.G., Hage, S.M., Kindaichi, M.M., & Bryant, R.M. (2007). Social justice and multicultural issues: implications for the practice and training of counselors and counseling psychologists. *Journal of Counseling & Development, 85*(1), 24–29.

Cook, A., Spinazzola, J., Ford, J., Lanktree, C., Blaustein, M., Cloitre, M., & van der Kolk, B. (2005). Complex trauma in children and adolescents. *Psychiatric Annals, 35,* 390–398.

Corey, G. (2004). *Theory and practice of group counseling* (6th ed.). Belmont, CA: Brooks/Cole-Thomson Learning.

Corey, G. (2012). *Theory and practice of group counseling* (8th ed.). Belmont, CA: Brooks/Cole.

Corey, G., Corey, M.S., & Callanan, P. (2011). *Issues and ethics in the helping professions* (8th ed.). Belmont, CA: Brooks/Cole.

Cowen, E., & Cruickshank, W. (1948). Group therapy with physically handicapped children II: Evaluation. *The Journal of Education Psychology, 39,* 281–297.

Cruickshank, W., & Cowen, E. (1948). Group therapy with physically handicapped children I: Report of study. *The Journal of Educational Psychology, 39,* 193–215.

Dahl, R.E., & Hariri, A.R. (2005). Lessons from G. Stanley Hall: Connecting new research in biological sciences to the study of adolescent development. *Journal of Research on Adolescence, 15*(4), 367–382.

Danger, S., & Landreth, G. (2005). Child-centered group play therapy with children with speech difficulties. *International Journal of Play Therapy, 14*, 81–102.

De Domenico, G.S. (1999). Group sandtray-worldplay: New dimensions in sandplay therapy. In D. Sweeney & L. Homeyer (Eds.), *Handbook of group play therapy: How to do it, how it works, whom it's best for* (pp. 215–233). San Francisco, CA: Jossey-Bass.

De Saint Exupery, A. (1943). *The little prince.* New York: Harcourt, Brace & World.

de Shazer, S. (1988). *Clues: Investigating solutions in brief therapy.* New York: Norton.

de Shazer, S., & Dolan, Y. (2007). *More than miracles: The state of the art of solution-focused brief therapy.* New York: Routledge.

Dempsey, D. (2010). Conceiving and negotiating reproductive relationships: Lesbians and gay men forming families with children. *Sociology, 44*(6), 1145–1162.

Douglas, C. (2008). Analytical psychotherapy. In R. Corsini & D. Wedding (Eds.), *Current psychotherapies* (8th ed., pp. 113–147). Belmont, CA: Thomson.

Drewes, A.A. (2009). *Blending play therapy with cognitive behavioral therapy: Evidence-based and other effective treatments and techniques.* Hoboken, NJ: John Wiley & Sons.

Drewes, A.A., Bratton, S.C., & Schaefer, C.E. (2011). *Integrative play therapy.* Hoboken, NJ: John Wiley & Sons.

Dulsky, S. (1942). Affect and intellect: An experimental study. *The Journal of General Psychology, 27*, 199–220.

Earls, M.K. (2011). The play factor: Effect of social skills group play therapy on adolescent African-American males. *Dissertation Abstracts International, A, 72.*

Education Trust (2009). *Education Watch State Report.* Texas: Education Trust. Available at www.edtrust.org/sites/edtrust.org/files/Texas_0.pdf

Elliot, D.B., & Simmons, T. (2011). *Marital events of Americans: 2009.* American Community Survey Reports. Washington, DC: United States Census Bureau.

Elliott, G., & Pumfrey, P. (1972). The effects of non-directive play therapy on some maladjusted boys. *Educational Research, 14*, 157–163.

Erford, B. (2011). *Group work: Processes and applications.* Upper Saddle River, NJ: Pearson Education.

Erikson, E.H. (1964). *Childhood and society* (2nd ed.). Oxford: W.W. Norton.

Fall, K., Holden, J., & Marquis, A. (2010). *Theoretical models of counseling and psychotherapy* (2nd ed.). New York: Routledge.

Fall, M., Balvanz, J., Johnson, L., & Nelson, L. (1999). The relationship of a play therapy intervention to self-efficacy and classroom learning. *Professional School Counseling, 2*, 194–204.

Fall, M., Navelski, L., & Welch, K. (2002). Outcomes of a play intervention for children identified for special education services. *International Journal of Play Therapy, 11*(2), 91–106.

Farahzadi, M., Bahramabadi, M., & Mohammadifar, M. (2011). Effectiveness of Gestalt play therapy in decreasing social phobia. *Journal of Iranian Psychologists, 7*, 387–395.

Fearnley, R. (2010). Death of a parent and the children's experience: Don't ignore the elephant in the room. *Journal of Interprofessional Care, 24*(4), 450–459.

Felix, E., Bond, D., & Shelby, J. (2006). Coping with disaster: Psychosocial interventions for children in international disaster relief. In C.E. Schaefer & H. Kaduson (Eds.), *Contemporary play therapy: Theory, research, and practice* (pp. 307–328). New York: Guilford Press.

Fischetti, B. (2010). Play therapy for anger management in the schools. In A. Drewes & C. Schaefer (Eds.), *School-based play therapy* (2nd ed., pp. 283–305). Hoboken, NJ: Wiley.

Fleming, L., & Snyder, W. (1947). Social and personal changes following nondirective group play therapy. *American Journal of Orthopsychiatry, 17*, 101–116.

Freud, A. (1946). *The psycho-analytical treatment of children*. New York: International Universities Press.

Freud, S. (1909/1955). *The case of "Little Hans" and the "Rat Man."* London: Hogarth Press.

Freud, S. (1949). *An outline of psychoanalysis*. New York: W.W. Norton & Co.

Gallo-Lopez, L. (2006). A creative play therapy approach to the group treatment of young sexually abused children. In H. Kaduson & C. Schaefer (Eds.), *Short-term play therapy for children* (2nd ed., pp. 245–272). New York: Guilford.

Gallo-Lopez, L., & Rubin, L. (2012). *Play-based interventions for children and adolescents with autism spectrum disorders*. New York: Routledge/Taylor & Francis.

Gallo-Lopez, L., & Schaefer, C.E. (2005). *Play therapy with adolescents*. Lanham, MD: Jason Aronson.

Gann, E. (2010). The effects of therapeutic hip hop activity groups on perception of self and social supports in at-risk urban adolescents. *Dissertation Abstracts International, 71.*

Garza, Y., & Bratton, S. (2005). School-based child-centered play therapy with Hispanic children: Outcomes and cultural considerations. *International Journal of Play Therapy, 14,* 51–71.

Gaskill, R.L., & Perry, B.D. (2012). Child sexual abuse, traumatic experiences, and their impact on the developing brain. In P. Goodyear-Brown (Ed.), *Handbook of child sexual abuse* (pp. 30–47). Hoboken, NJ: John Wiley & Sons.

Gaulden, G. (1975). Developmental-play group counseling with early primary grade students exhibiting behavioral problems (Doctoral dissertation, North Texas State University, 1975). *Dissertation Abstracts International, 36,* 2628.

Gendler, M. (1986). Group puppetry with school-age children: Rationale, procedure, and therapeutic implications. *The Arts in Psychotherapy, 13,* 45–52.

Gil, E. (1994). *Play in family therapy*. New York: Guilford Press.

Gil, E. (2006). *Helping abused and traumatized children: Integrating directive and nondirective approaches*. New York: Guilford Press.

Gil, E. (2011). *Helping abused and traumatized children: Integrating directive and nondirective approaches*. New York: Guildford.

Gil, E., & Drewes, A.A. (2005). *Cultural issues in play therapy*. New York: Guilford Press.

Ginott, H. (1958). Play group therapy: A theoretical framework. *International Journal of Group Psychotherapy, 8*(4), 410–418.

Ginott, H. (1961). *Group psychotherapy with children: The theory and practice of play therapy*. New York: McGraw-Hill.

Ginott, H. (1982). Group play therapy with children. In G. Landreth (Ed.), *Play therapy: Dynamics of the process of counseling with children* (pp. 327–341). Springfield, IL: Charles C. Thomas.

Ginott, H. (1999) Play group therapy: A theoretical framework. In D. Sweeney & L. Homeyer (Eds.), *Handbook of group play therapy: How to do it, how it works, whom it's best for* (pp. 15–23). San Francisco: Jossey-Bass. (Original work published 1948).

Gladding, S. (2012). *Group work: A counseling specialty* (6th ed.). Upper Saddle River, NJ: Pearson.

Glover, G. (2005). Musings on working with Native American children in play therapy. In E. Gil & A.A. Drewes (Eds.), *Cultural issues in play therapy* (pp. 168–179). New York: Guilford Press.

Goldberg, A.E., Smith, J.Z., & Perry-Jenkins, M. (2012). The division of labor in lesbian, gay, and heterosexual new adoptive parents. *Journal of Marriage and Family, 74*(4), 812–828.

Goldman, L. (2006). Best practice grief work with students in schools. In C. Franklin, M.B. Harris, & P. Allen-Meares (Eds.) *The school services sourcebook: A guide for school based professionals* (pp. 567–575). Oxford: Oxford University Press.

Gould, M. (1980). The effect of short-term intervention play therapy on the self-concept of selected elementary pupils (Doctoral dissertation, Florida Institute of Technology, 1980). *Dissertation Abstracts International, 41*, 1090.

Green, E.J. (2007). The crisis of family separation following traumatic mass destruction: Jungian analytical play therapy in the aftermath of hurricane Katrina. In N.B. Webb (Ed.), *Play therapy with children in crisis: Individual, group, and family treatment* (3rd ed., pp. 368–388). New York: The Guilford Press.

Green, E. (2009). Jungian analytical play therapy. In K. O'Connor & L. Braverman (Eds.), *Play therapy theory and practice: Comparing theories and techniques* (2nd ed., pp. 83–121). Hoboken, NJ: Wiley.

Green, E., Crenshaw, D., & Drewes, A. (October 13, 2011). *Depth approaches to foster resilience in children following trauma.* A half-day workshop presented at the Annual Association for Play Therapy International Conference, Sacramento, CA.

Green, E.J., McCollum, V.C., & Hays, D. (2008). Teaching advocacy counseling within a social justice framework: Implications for school counselors and educators. *Journal of Social Action in Counseling and Psychology, 1*(2), 14–30.

Guha-Sapir, D., Vos, F., Below, R., & Ponserre, S. (2012). *Annual disaster statistical review 2011: the numbers and trends.* Brussels: CRED.

Hadley, S., & Yancy, G. (2012). *Therapeutic uses of rap and hip-hop.* New York: Routledge.

Haine, R.A., Ayers, T.S., Sandler, I.N., & Wolchik, S.A. (2008). Evidence-based practices for parentally bereaved children and their families. *Professional Psychology: Research and Practice, 39*(2), 113–121.

Hall, G.S. (1904). *Adolescence. Its psychology and its relations to physiology, anthropology, sociology, sex, crime, religion, and education.* New York: Appleton.

Hansen, S. (2006). An expressive arts therapy model with groups for post-traumatic stress disorder. In L. Carey (Ed.), *Expressive and creative arts methods for trauma survivors* (pp. 73–91). London: Jessica Kingsley.

Haworth, M. (1994). *Child psychotherapy: Practice and theory.* Northvale, NJ: Aronson.

Herman, J. (1992). *Trauma and recovery: The aftermath of violence—from domestic abuse to political terror.* New York: Basic Books.

Hinds, S. (2005). Play therapy in the African American "Village". In E. Gil & A.A. Drewes (Eds.), *Cultural issues in play therapy* (pp. 115–147). New York: Guilford Press.

Holmberg, J.R., Benedict, H.E., & Hynan, L.S. (1998). Gender differences in children's play therapy themes: Comparisons of children with a history of attachment disturbance or exposure to violence. *International Journal of Play Therapy, 7*(2), 67–92.

Holmes, M. (2000). *A terrible thing happened—A story for children who witnessed violence or trauma.* Washington, DC: Magination Press.

Homeyer, L., & Sweeney, D. (2011). *Sandtray therapy: A practical manual* (2nd ed.). New York: Routledge.

Hopkins, S., Huici, V., & Bermudez, D. (2005). Therapeutic play with Hispanic clients. In E. Gil & A.A. Drewes (Eds.), *Cultural issues in play therapy* (pp. 148–167). New York: Guilford Press.

House, R. (1970). The effects of nondirective group play therapy upon the sociometric status and self-concept of selected second grade children (Doctoral dissertation, Oregon State University, 1970). *Dissertation Abstracts International, 31*, 2684.

Hume, K. (1967). A counseling service project for grades one through four. (Doctoral dissertation, Boston University, 1967). *Dissertation Abstracts International, 27*(12A), 4130.

Hunter, L. (2006). Group sandtray play therapy. In H. Kaduson & C. Schaefer (Eds.), *Short-term play therapy for children* (2nd ed., pp. 273–303). New York: Guilford Press.

Inhelder, B., Piaget, J., Parsons, A., & Milgram, S. (1958). *The growth of logical thinking: From childhood to adolescence*. New York, NY: Basic Books.

Irwin, E. (2000). The use of a puppet interview to understand children. In K. Gitlin-Weiner, A. Sandgrund & C. Schaefer (Eds.), *Play diagnosis and assessment* (2nd ed., pp. 682–703). New York: Wiley.

Irwin, E., & Malloy, E. (1994). Family puppet interview. In C. Schaefer & L. Carey (Eds.), *Family play therapy* (pp. 21–48). Lanham, MD: Jason Aronson.

Ivey, A., D'Andrea, M., Ivey, M., & Simek-Morgan, L. (2006). *Theories of counseling and psychotherapy: A multicultural perspective* (6th ed.). Boston, MA: Allyn & Bacon.

Jacobs, E., Masson, R., Harvill, R., & Schimmel. (2012). *Group counseling: Strategies and skills* (7th ed.). Belmont, CA: Brooks/Cole.

Jalali, S., & Molavi, H. (2011). The effect of play therapy on separation anxiety disorder in children. *Journal of Psychology, 14*, 370–382.

James, W. (1891). *The principles of psychology, Volume I*. London: Macmillan & Co.

Jaycox, L.H., Cohen, J.A., Mannarino, A.P., Walker, D.W., Langley, A.K., Gegenheimer, K.L., & Schonlau, M. (2010). Children's mental health care following Hurricane Katrina: A field trial of trauma-focused psychotherapies. *Journal of Traumatic Stress, 23*(2), 223–231.

Johnson, L. (2012). *Kick-start your class: Academic icebreakers to engage students*. San Francisco, CA: Jossey Bass.

Jones, R.T., Fletcher, K., & Ribbe, D.R. (2002). *Child's Reaction to Traumatic Events Scale-Revised (CRTES-R): A self-report traumatic stress measure*. Blackburg, VA: Author.

Kaduson, H.G., & Schaefer, C.E. (1997). *101 favorite play therapy techniques*. Lanham, MD: Jason Aronson.

Kaduson, H., & Schaefer, C. (2001). *101 more favorite play therapy techniques*. Lanham, MD: Jason Aronson.

Kaduson, H., & Schaefer, C. (Eds.) (2004). *101 more favorite play therapy techniques*. Lanham, MD: Rowman & Littlefield.

Kalff, D. (1980). *Sandplay, a psychotherapeutic approach to the psyche*. Santa Monica, CA: Sigo Press.

Kao, S. (2005). Play therapy with Asian children. In E. Gil & A.A. Drewes (Eds.), *Cultural issues in play therapy* (pp. 180–193). New York: Guilford Press.

Kao, S., & Landreth, G.L. (2001). Play therapy with Chinese children: Needed modifications. In G.L. Landreth (Ed.), *Innovations in play therapy: Issues, process, and special populations* (pp. 43–49). New York: Brunner-Routledge.

Kenney-Noziska, S., Schaefer, C., & Homeyer, L. (2012). Beyond directive or nondirective: Moving the conversation forward. *International Journal of Play Therapy, 21*(4), 244–252.

Kestly, T. (2010). Group sandplay in elementary schools. In A. Drewes, L. Carey, & C. Schaefer (Eds.), *School-based play therapy* (2nd ed., pp. 257–281). Hoboken, NJ: John Wiley & Sons.

Kirwin, K.M., & Hamrin, V. (2005). Decreasing the risk of complicated bereavement and future psychiatric disorders in children. *Journal of Child and Adolescent Psychiatric Nursing, 18*(2), 62–78.

Klein, M. (1929). Personification in the play of children. *International Journal of Psychoanalysis, 10*, 193–204.

Klein, M. (1975/1932). *The psycho-analysis of children*. New York: Delacorte Press.

Knell, S. (1993). *Cognitive-behavioral play therapy*. Northvale, NJ: Jason Aronson.

Knell, S. (1994). Cognitive behavioral play therapy. In K. O'Connor & C. Schaefer (Eds.), *Handbook of play therapy: Advances and innovations* (Vol. 2, pp. 111–142). New York: Wiley.

Knell, S. (2009). Cognitive-behavioral play therapy. In K. O'Connor & L. Braverman (Eds.), *Play therapy theory and practice: Comparing theories and techniques* (2nd ed., pp. 203–236). Hoboken, NJ: Wiley.

Knell, S. (2011). Cognitive-behavioral play therapy. In C. Schaefer (Ed.), *Foundations of play therapy* (2nd ed., pp. 313–328). Hoboken, NJ: John Wiley & Sons.

Knell, S., & Beck, K. (2000). The puppet sentence completion task. In K. Gitlin-Weiner, A. Sandgrund, & C. Schaefer (Eds.), *Play diagnosis and assessment* (2nd ed., pp. 704–721). New York: Wiley.

Knell, S., & Dasari, M. (2011). Cognitive-behavioral play therapy. In S. Russ & L. Niec (Eds.), *Play in clinical practice: Evidence-based approaches* (pp. 236–263). New York: Guilford.

Kohlberg, L. (1981). *Essays on moral development: Vol. 1, The philosophy of moral development.* San Francisco, CA: Harper & Row.

Kohlberg, L., & Gilligan, C. (1972). The adolescent as a philosopher: The discovery of the self in a post-conventional world (pp. 148–155). In J. Kagan & R. Coles (Eds.), *Twelve to sixteen: Early adolescence.* Oxford: W.W. Norton.

Kotchick, B.A., & Forehand, R. (2002). Putting parenting in perspective: A discussion of the contextual factors that shape parenting practices. *Journal of Child and Family Studies, 11*(3), 255–269.

Kottman, T. (1999). Group applications of Adlerian play therapy. In D. Sweeney & L. Homeyer (Eds.), *The handbook of group play therapy: How to do it, how it works, whom it's best for* (pp. 65–85). San Francisco, CA: Jossey-Bass.

Kottman, T. (2003). *Partners in play: An Adlerian approach to play therapy* (2nd ed.). Alexandria, VA: American Counseling Association.

Kottman, T. (2009). Adlerian play therapy. In K. O'Connor & L. Braverman (Eds.), *Play therapy theory and practice: Comparing theories and techniques* (2nd ed., pp. 237–282). Hoboken, NJ: Wiley.

Kottman, T. (2010). *Play therapy: Basics and beyond* (2nd ed.). Alexandria, VA: American Counseling Association.

Kovacs, M. (1982). *Children's Depression Inventory.* Pittsburgh: Western Psychiatric Institute and Clinic.

Kramer, E. (1993). *Art as therapy with children.* Chicago, IL: Magnolia Street.

Kronenberg, M.E., Hansel, T., Brennan, A.M., Osofsky, H.J., Osofsky, J.D., & Lawrason, B. (2010). Children of Katrina: Lessons learned about postdisaster symptoms and recovery patterns. *Child Development, 81*(4), 1241–1259.

La Greca, A. (2008). Interventions for posttraumatic stress in children and adolescents following natural disasters and acts of terrorism. In R.C. Steele, T.D. Elkin, & M.C. Roberts (Eds.), *Handbook of evidence-based therapies for children and adolescents: Bridging science and practice* (pp. 121–141). New York: Springer Science.

La Greca, A.M., & Silverman, W.K. (2009). Treatment and prevention of posttraumatic stress reactions in children and adolescents exposed to disasters and terrorism: What is the evidence? *Child Development Perspectives, 3*(1), 4–10.

La Greca, A.M., Sevin, S., & Sevin, E. (2001). *Helping America cope: A guide for parents and children in the aftermath of the September 11th national disaster.* Miami, FL: Sevendippity.

La Greca, A.M., Sevin, S., & Sevin, E. (2005). *After the storm.* Miami, FL: Sevendippity.

La Greca, A.M., Silverman, W.K., Vernberg, E.M., & Prinstein, M. (1996). Symptoms of posttraumatic stress after Hurricane Andrew: A prospective study. *Journal of Consulting and Clinical Psychology, 64*, 712–723.

La Greca, A.M., Silverman, W.K., Lai, B., & Jaccard, J. (2010). Hurricane-related exposure experiences and stressors, other life events, and social support: Concurrent and prospective impact on children's persistent posttraumatic stress symptoms. *Journal of Consulting and Clinical Psychology,* doi: 10.1037/a0020775.

La Greca, A.M., Silverman, W.K., Vernberg, E.M., & Roberts, M.C. (2002). *Helping children cope with disasters and terrorism.* Washington, DC: American Psychological Association Press.

Lambert, S., LeBlanc, M., Mullen, J., Ray, D., Baggerly, J., White, J., & Kaplan, D. (2005). Learning more about those who play in session: The national play therapy in counseling practices project. *Journal of Counseling & Development, 85,* 42–46.

Landgarten, H.B. (1987). *Family art psychotherapy: A clinical guide and casebook.* New York: Brunner/Mazel.

Landreth, G.L. (2012). *Play therapy: The art of relationship* (3rd ed.). New York: Routledge/Taylor & Francis.

Landreth, G., & Sweeney, D. (1999). The freedom to be: Child-centered group play therapy. In D. Sweeney & L. Homeyer (Eds.), *The handbook of group play therapy: How to do it, how it works, whom it's best for* (pp. 39–64). San Francisco, CA: Jossey-Bass.

Lasky, G., & Riva, M. (2006). Confidentiality and privileged communication in group psychotherapy. *International Journal of Group Psychotherapy, 56*(4), 455–476.

Le Vieux, J. (1999). Group play therapy with grieving children. In D.S. Sweeney & L. Homeyer (Eds.), *The handbook of group play therapy: How to do it, how it works, whom* it's best for (pp. 375–388). San Francisco, CA: Jossey-Bass.

LeBlanc, M., & Ritchie, M. (2001). A meta-analysis of play therapy outcomes. *Counselling Psychology Quarterly, 14,* 149–163.

Lee, A. (2009). Psychoanalytic play therapy. In K. O'Connor & L. Braverman (Eds.), *Play therapy theory and practice: Comparing theories and techniques* (pp. 25–81). Hoboken, NJ: John Wiley & Sons.

Lev, E.L. (1983). An activity therapy group with children in an in-patient psychiatric setting. *Psychiatric Quaterly, 55,* 55–64.

Life Center of the Suncoast Inc. (2005). *TLC articles: Lean on me.* Retrieved from www.lifecenteroftampa.org/sheryleart.htm

Lowenfeld, M. (1979). *The world technique.* London: George Allen & Unwin.

Lowenstein, L. (Ed.) (2008). *Assessment and treatment activities for children, adolescents, and families: Practitioners share their most effective techniques.* Toronto: Champion Press.

Lowenstein, L. (Ed.) (2010). *Creative family therapy techniques: Play, art, and expressive activities to engage children in family sessions.* Toronto: Champion Press.

Ludlow, W., & Williams, M. (2006). Short-term group play therapy for children whose parents are divorcing. In H. Kaduson & C. Schaefer (Eds.), *Short-term play therapy for children* (2nd ed., pp. 304–335). New York: Guilford.

Lyons, J.S., Griffin, E., Fazio, M., & Lyons, M.B. (1999). *Child and adolescent needs and strengths: An information integration tool for children and adolescents with mental health challenges (CANS-MH), manual.* Chicago, IL: Buddin Praed Foundation.

Mahmoudi-Gharaei, J., Bina, M., Yasami, M., Emami, A., & Naderi, F. (2006). Group play therapy effect on Bam earthquake related emotional and behavioral symptoms in preschool children: A before-after trial. *Iranian Journal of Pediatrics, 16,* 137–142.

Malchiodi, C.A. (2005). *Expressive therapies.* New York: Guilford Press.

Malchiodi, C.A. (2008). *Creative interventions with traumatized children.* New York: Guilford Press.

Massat, C., Moses, H., & Ornstein, E. (2008). Grief and loss in schools: A perspective for school social workers. *School Social Work Journal, 33*(1), 80–96.

McNiff, S. (2009). *Integrating the arts in therapy: History, theory, and practice.* Springfield, IL: Charles C. Thomas.

McRae, M.B., & Short, E.L. (2010). *Racial and cultural dynamics in group and organizational life: Crossing boundaries.* Thousand Oaks, CA: Sage.

Measelle, J., Ablow, J., Cowan, P., & Cowan, C. (1998). Assessing young children's views of their academic, social, and emotional lives: An evaluation of the self-perception scales of the Berkeley Puppet Interview. *Child Development, 69,* 1556–1576.

Mehlman, B. (1953). Group play therapy with mentally retarded children. *Journal of Abnormal and Social Psychology, 48*, 53–60.

Mosak, H., & Maniacci, M. (2008). Adlerian psychotherapy. In R. Corsini & D. Wedding (Eds.), *Current psychotherapies* (8th ed., pp. 67–112). Belmont, CA: Thomson.

Moulin, E. (1970). The effects of client-centered group counseling using play media on the intelligence, achievement, and psycholinguistic abilities of underachieving primary school children. *Elementary School Guidance and Counseling, 5*, 85–98.

Moustakas, C. (1959). *Psychotherapy with children: The living relationship*. New York: Harper & Row.

Mundy, L. (1957). Therapy with physically and mentally handicapped children in a mental deficiency hospital. *Journal of Clinical Psychology, 13*, 3–9.

Muro, J., Ray, D., Schottelkorb, A., Smith, M., & Blanco, P. (2006). Quantitative analysis of long term play therapy. *International Journal of Play Therapy, 15*, 35–58.

Naderi, F., Heidarie, A., Bouron, L., & Asgari, P. (2010). The efficacy of play therapy on ADHD, anxiety, and social maturity in 8 to 12 years aged clientele children of Ahwaz metropolitan counseling clinics. *Journal of Applied Sciences, 10*, 189–195.

Nash, J., & Schaefer, C. (2011). Play therapy: Basic concepts and practices. In C. Schaefer (Ed.), *Foundations of play therapy* (2nd ed., pp. 3–14). Hoboken, NJ: John Wiley & Sons.

National Commission on Children and Disasters. (2010). *2010 Report to the President and Congress*. AHRQ Publication No. 10-M037. Rockville, MD: Agency for Healthcare Research and Quality.

National Institute on Drug Abuse. (2012). *Monitoring the future 2012: Teen drug use*. Washington, DC: National Institute of Health.

Newcomer, B., & Morrison, T. (1974). Play therapy with institutionalized mentally retarded children. *American Journal of Mental Deficiency, 78*, 727–733.

Nikulina, V., Widom, C., & Czaja, S. (2011). The role of childhood neglect and childhood poverty in predicting mental health, academic achievement and crime in adulthood. *American Journal of Community Psychology, 48*(3–4), 309–321.

Nims, D. (2011). Solution-focused play therapy: Helping children and families find solutions. In C. Schaefer (Ed.), *Foundations of play therapy* (2nd ed., pp. 297–312). Hoboken, NJ: John Wiley & Sons.

Norton, C., & Norton, B. (2002). *Reaching children through play therapy: An experiential approach* (2nd ed.). Denver, CO: White Apple Press.

Oaklander, V. (1988). *Windows to our children*. Highland, NY: The Gestalt Journal Press.

Oaklander, V. (1999). Group play therapy from a Gestalt therapy perspective. In D. Sweeney & L. Homeyer (Eds.), *The handbook of group play therapy: How to do it, how it works, whom it's best for* (pp. 162–175). San Francisco, CA: Jossey-Bass.

O'Connor, K. (1983). The color-your-life technique. In C. Schaefer & K. O'Connor (Eds.), *Handbook of play therapy* (pp. 251–258). New York: Wiley.

O'Connor, K. (1994). Ecosystemic play therapy. In K. O'Connor & C. Schaefer (Eds.). *Handbook of play therapy: Advances and innovations* (Vol. 2, pp. 61–84). New York: Wiley.

O'Connor, K. (1999). Child, protector, confidant: Structured group Ecosystemic play therapy. In D. Sweeney & L. Homeyer (Eds.), *The handbook of group play therapy: How to do it, how it works, whom it's best for* (pp. 105–138). San Francisco, CA: Jossey-Bass.

O'Connor, K. (2000). *The play therapy primer* (2nd ed.). New York: John Wiley & Sons.

O'Connor, K. (2009). Ecosystemic play therapy. In K. O'Connor & L. Braverman (Eds.), *Play therapy theory and practice: Comparing theories and techniques* (pp. 367–447). Hoboken, NJ: John Wiley & Sons.

O'Connor, K., & Ammen, S. (1997). *Play therapy treatment planning and interventions: The Ecosystemic model and workbook*. San Diego, CA: Academic Press.

Our Military Kids. (2013). *White paper on our military kids.* Retrieved from www.ourmili-tarykids.org/wp-content/uploads/2011/03/White-Paper-Our-Military-Kids.pdf

Pablo Picasso. (n.d.). BrainyQuote.com. Retrieved January 18, 2013 from www.brainyquote.com/quotes/quotes/p/pablopicas102627.html

Packman, J., & Bratton, S.C. (2003). A school-based group play/activity therapy intervention with learning disabled preadolescents exhibiting behavior problems. *International Journal of Play Therapy, 12*(2), 7–29.

Pane, J., McCaffrey, D.F., Kalra, N., & Zhou, A. (2008). Effects of student displacement in Louisiana during the first academic year after the hurricanes of 2005. *Journal of Education for Children Placed at Risk, 13*(2), 168–211.

Paone, T.R., Packman, J., Maddux, C., & Rothman, T. (2008). A school-based group activity therapy intervention with at-risk high school students as it relates to their moral reasoning. *International Journal of Play Therapy, 17*(2), 122–137.

Parham, T.A., White, J.L., & Ajamu, A. (2000). *The psychology of Blacks: An African centered perspective.* Upper Saddle River, NJ: Prentice-Hall.

Parsons, R. (2007). *Counseling strategies that work! Evidence-based interventions for school counselors.* Boston, MA: Pearson Education.

Pelham, L. (1972). Self-directive play therapy with socially immature kindergarten students (Doctoral dissertation, University of Northern Colorado, 1971). *Dissertation Abstracts International, 32*, 3798.

Perez, C. (1987). A comparison of group play therapy and individual play therapy for sexually abused children (Doctoral dissertation, University of Northern Colorado, 1987). *Dissertation Abstracts International, 48*, 3079.

Perry, B.D. (2006). Applying principles of neurodevelopment to clinical work with maltreated and traumatized children: The neurosequential model of therapeutics. In N. Webb (Ed.), *Working with traumatized youth in child welfare* (pp. 27–52). New York: Guilford Press.

Perry, B.D. (2009). Examining child maltreatment through a neurodevelopmental lens: Clinical application of the neurosequential model of therapeutics. *Journal of Loss and Trauma, 14*, 240–255.

Perry, B., Pollard, R., Blakely, T., Baker, W., & Vigilante, D. (1995). Childhood trauma, the neurobiological adaptation and "use-dependent" development of the brain: How "states become traits." *Infant Mental Health Journal, 26*(4), 271–291.

Piaget, J. (1962). The stages of the intellectual development of the child. *Bulletin of the Menninger Clinic, 26*, 120–128.

Pincus, D., Chase, R., Chow, C., Weiner, C., & Pian, J. (2011). Integrating play into cognitive-behavioral therapy for child anxiety disorders. In S. Russ & L. Niec (Eds.), *Play in clinical practice: Evidence-based approaches* (pp. 218–235). New York: Guilford.

Post Sprunk, T. (2010). Beach ball game. In L. Lowenstein (Ed.), *Creative family therapy techniques: Play, art, and expressive activities to engage children in family sessions* (pp. 9–12). Toronto: Champion Press.

Prior, S. (1996). *Object relations in severe trauma: Psychotherapy with sexually abused children.* Northvale, NJ: Jason Aronson.

Prout, S., & Prout, H.T. (2007). Ethical and legal issues in psychological interventions with children and adolescents. In H.T. Prout & D. Brown (Eds.), *Counseling and psychotherapy with children and adolescents: Theory and practice for school and clinical settings* (4th ed., pp. 32–63). Hoboken, NJ: John Wiley & Sons.

Pynoos, R., Rodriguez, N., Steinberg, A., Stuber, M., & Frederick, C. (1998). *UCLA PTSD Index for DSM-IV.*

Ragsdale, S., & Saylor, A. (2007). *Great group games: 175 boredom-busting, zero-prep team builders for all ages.* Minneapolis, MN: Search Institute Press.

Ray, D. (2007). Two counseling interventions to reduce teacher-child relationship stress. *Professional School Counseling, 10,* 428–440.

Ray, D. (2011). *Advanced play therapy: Essential conditions, knowledge, and skills for child practice.* New York: Routledge.

Ray, D., Armstrong, S., Balkin, R., & Jayne, K. (in review). *Child centered play therapy in the schools: Review and meta-analysis.*

Ray, D., Blanco, P., Sullivan, J., & Holliman, R. (2009). Child centered play therapy with aggressive children. *International Journal of Play Therapy, 18,* 162–175.

Ray, D., Schottelkorb, A., & Tsai, M. (2007). Play therapy with children exhibiting symptoms of attention deficit hyperactivity disorder. *International Journal of Play Therapy, 16,* 95–111.

Reddy, L. (2012). *Group play interventions for children: Strategies for teaching prosocial skills.* Washington, DC: American Psychological Association.

Remley, T., & Herlihy, B. (2005). *Ethical, legal, and professional issues in counseling* (2nd ed.). Upper Saddle River, NJ: Pearson Education.

Reynolds, C.R., & Richmond, B.O. (1985). *Revised Children's Manifest Anxiety Scale.* RCMAS Manual. Los Angeles: Western Psychological Services.

Riviere, S. (2005). Play therapy techniques to engage adolescents. In L. Gallo-Lopez & C.E. Schaefer (Eds.), *Play therapy with adolescents* (pp. 121–142). Lanham, MD: Jason Aronson.

Robles, R. (2006). Culturally competent play therapy with the Mexican American child and family. In C.E. Schaefer & H. Kaduson (Eds.), *Contemporary play therapy: Theory, research, and practice* (pp. 238–269). New York: Guilford Press.

Rogers, C. (1951). *Client-centered therapy: Its current practice, implications and theory.* Boston: Houghton Mifflin.

Rogers, C. (1957). The necessary and sufficient conditions of therapeutic personality change. *Journal of Consulting Psychology, 21*(2), 95–103.

Rogers, C. (1970). *Carl Rogers on encounter groups.* New York: Harper & Row.

Rollins, J. (2008). Arts for children in hospitals: Helping to put the "art" back in medicine. In B. Warren (Ed.), *Using the creative arts in therapy and healthcare: A practical introduction* (3rd ed., pp. 181–195). New York: Routledge/Taylor & Francis.

Roos, B.M., & Jones, S.A. (1982). Working with girls experiencing loss: An application of activity group therapy in a multiethnic community. *Social Work with Groups: A Journal of Community and Clinical Practice, 5,* 35–49.

Rosenfeld, L.B., Caye, J.S., Ayalon, O., & Lahad, M. (2005). *When their world falls apart: Helping families and children manage the effects of disasters.* Washington, DC: NASW Press.

Ross, P. (2000). The family puppet technique for assessing parent–child and family interaction patterns. In K. Gitlin-Weiner, A. Sandgrund, & C. Schaefer (Eds.), *Play diagnosis and assessment* (2nd ed., pp. 672–681). New York: Wiley.

Rubin, J. (2010). *Introduction to art therapy: Sources and resources.* New York: Routledge/Taylor & Francis.

Rubin, J.A. (2011). *The art of art therapy: What every art therapist needs to know.* New York: Routledge/Taylor & Francis.

Saigh, P.A. (2004). *A structural interview for diagnosing Posttraumatic Stress Disorder: Children's PTSD Inventory.* San Antonio, TX: PsychCorp.

Sales, B., DeKraai, M., Hall, S., & Duvall, J. (2008). Child therapy and the law. In R. Morris & T. Kratochwill (Eds.), *The practice of child therapy* (4th ed., pp. 519–542). New York: Routledge.

Salloum, A., Garside, L.W., Irwin, C., Anderson, A.D., & Francois, A.H. (2009). Grief and trauma group therapy for children after Hurricane Katrina. *Social Work with Groups: A Journal of Community and Clinical Practice, 32*(1–2), 64–79.

Schaefer, C., & Reid, S. (Eds.). (2001) *Game Play: Therapeutic Use of Childhood Games* (2nd ed.). New York: Wiley.

Scheeringa, M.S. (2005). *Disaster Experiences Questionnaire*. Unpublished measure. New Orleans, LA: Tulane University.

Scheidlinger, S. (1977). Group therapy for latency-age children: A bird's eye view. *Journal of Clinical Child Psychology, 6*(1), 40–43.

Schiffer, A. (1966). The effectiveness of group play therapy as assessed by specific changes in a child's peer relations. *Dissertation Abstracts International, 27B*, 972.

Schiffer, M. (1952). Permissiveness versus sanction in activity group therapy. *International Journal of Group Psychotherapy, 2*, 225–261.

Schiffer, M. (1977). Activity group therapy: Implications in community agency practice. *Group, 1*(4), 211–221.

Schoen, A., Burgoyne, M., & Schoen, S. (2004). Are the developmental needs of children in America adequately addressed during the grief process? *Journal of Instructional Psychology, 31*(2), 143–148.

Schoon, I., Jones, E., Cheng, H., & Maughan, B. (2012). Family hardship, family instability, and cognitive development. *Journal of Epidemiology and Community Health, 66*(8), 716–722.

Schottelkorb, A., & Ray, D. (2009). ADHD symptom reduction in elementary students: A single case effectiveness design. *Professional School Counseling, 13*, 11–22.

Schumann, B. (2010). Effectiveness of child centered play therapy for children referred for aggression. In J. Baggerly, D. Ray, & S. Bratton (Eds.), *Child centered play therapy research: The evidence base for effective practice* (pp. 193–208). Hoboken, NJ: Wiley.

Seeman, J., & Edwards, B. (1954). A therapeutic approach to reading difficulties. *Journal of Consulting Psychology, 18*, 451–453.

Shelby, J., & Felix, E. (2005). Posttraumatic play therapy: The need for an integrated model of directive and nondirective approaches. In L. Reddy, T. Files-Hall, & C. Schaefer (Eds.), *Empirically based play interventions for children* (pp. 79–103). Washington, DC: American Psychological Association.

Shen, Y. (2002). Short-term group play therapy with Chinese earthquake victims: Effects on anxiety, depression, and adjustment. *International Journal of Play Therapy, 11*, 43–63.

Shephard, C. (1998). *Brave Bart: A story for traumatized and grieving children*. Clinton Township, MI: Trauma and Loss in Children.

Shmukler, D., & Naveh, I. (1984). Structured vs. unstructured play training with economically disadvantaged pre-schoolers. *Imagination, Cognition and Personality, 4*, 293–304.

Siegel, C. (1970). The effectiveness of play therapy with other modalities in the treatment of children with learning disabilities (Doctoral dissertation, Boston University, 1970). *Dissertation Abstracts International, 48*, 2112.

Slack, K., Holl, J.L., McDaniel, M., Yoo, J., & Bolger, K. (2004). Understanding the risks of child neglect: An exploration of poverty and parenting characteristics. *Child Maltreatment, 9*(4), 395–408.

Slavson, S. (1943). *Introduction to group therapy*. New York: The Commonwealth Fund.

Slavson, S. (1944). Some elements in activity group therapy. *American Journal of Orthopsychiatry, 14*, 578–588.

Slavson, S. (1945). Treatment of withdrawal through group therapy. *American Journal of Orthopsychiatry, 15*, 681–689.

Slavson, S. (1948). Play group therapy for young children. *Nervous Child, 7*, 318–327.

Slavson, S. (1999). Play group therapy for young children. In D. Sweeney & L. Homeyer (Eds.), *Handbook of group play therapy: How to do it, how it works, whom it's best for* (pp. 24–35). San Francisco: Jossey-Bass. (Original work published 1948.)

Slavson, S., & Schiffer, M. (1975). *Group psychotherapies for children: A textbook*. New York: International Universities Press.

Smith, D., & Smith, N.R. (1999). Relational activity play therapy group: A "stopping off place" for children on their journey to maturity. In D. Sweeney & L. Homeyer (Eds.), *Handbook of group play therapy: How to do it, how it works, whom it's best for* (pp. 234–266). San Francisco: Jossey-Bass. (Original work published 1948.)

Sokoloff, M. (1959). A comparison of gains in communicative skills, resulting from group play therapy and individual speech therapy, among a group of non-severely dysarthric, speech handicapped cerebral palsied children (Doctoral dissertation, New York University, 1959). *Dissertation Abstracts International, 20,* 803.

Speier, A. (2000). *Psychosocial issues for children and adolescents in disasters* (2nd ed.). Rockville, MD: Center for Mental Health Services, Substance Abuse and Mental Health Services Administration. Retrieved from store.samhsa.gov/product/Psychosocial-Issues-for-Children-and-Adolescents-in-Disasters/ADM86-1070R

Sue, D.W., Bernier, J.E., Durran, A., Feinberg, L., Pedersen, P., Smith, E.J., & Vasquez-Nuttall, E. (1982). Position paper: Cross-cultural counseling competencies. *The Counseling Psychologist,* 10, 45–52.

Sweeney, D. (1997). *Counseling children through the world of play.* Eugene, OR: Wipf and Stock.

Sweeney, D. (2001). Legal and ethical issues in play therapy. In G. Landreth (Ed.), *Innovations in play therapy: Issues, process, and special populations* (pp. 65–82). Philadelphia, PA: Brunner-Routledge.

Sweeney, D. (2011a). Group play therapy. In C. Schaefer (Ed.), *Foundations of play therapy* (2nd ed., pp. 227–252). Hoboken, NJ: John Wiley & Sons.

Sweeney, D. (2011b). Integration of sandtray therapy and solution-focused techniques for treating noncompliant youth. In A. Drewes, S. Bratton, & C. Schaefer (Eds.), *Integrative play therapy* (pp. 61–74). Hoboken, NJ: John Wiley & Sons.

Sweeney, D., & Homeyer, L. (1999). *Handbook of group play therapy: How to do it, how it works, whom it's best for.* San Francisco, CA: Jossey-Bass.

Sweeney, D., & Homeyer, L. (2009). Sandtray therapy. In A. Drewes (Ed.), *Effectively blending play therapy and cognitive behavioral therapy: A convergent approach* (pp. 297–318). Hoboken, NJ: John Wiley & Sons.

Tabin, J. (2005). Transitional objects in play therapy with adolescents. In L. Gallo-Lopez & C.E. Schaefer (Eds.), *Play therapy with adolescents* (pp. 68–80). Lanham, MD: Jason Aronson.

Tan, T., & Baggerly, J. (2009). Behavioral adjustment of adopted Chinese girls in single-mother, lesbian-couple, and heterosexual-couple households. *Adoption Quarterly, 12*(3–4), 171–186.

Tasker, F., & Golombok, S. (1997). *Growing up in a lesbian family: Effects on child development.* New York: Guilford Press.

Taylor, A., & Abell, S.C. (2005). The use of poetry in play therapy with adolescents. In L. Gallo-Lopez & C.E. Schaefer (Eds.), *Play therapy with adolescents* (pp. 143–158). Lanham, MD: Jason Aronson.

Terr, L. (1990). *Too scared to cry: Psychic trauma in childhood.* New York: Basic Books.

The Theraplay® Institute (2005). *Theraplay® Group Activities: 85 fun Theraplay® for groups of children.* Wilmette, IL: The Theraplay® Institute.

The Theraplay® Institute (2006). *Theraplay group activities flip book.* Evanston, IL: The Theraplay Institute.

Thomas, P. (2001). *I miss you. A first look at death.* Hauppauge, NY: Barron's Educational Series.

Thomas, R.V., & Pender, D. (2008). Association for specialists in group work: Best practice guidelines 2007 revisions. *The Journal for Specialists in Group Work, 33*(2), 111–117.

Thombs, M., & Muro, J. (1973). Group counseling and the sociometric status of second grade children. *Elementary School Guidance and Counseling, 7,* 194–197.

Troester, J.D. (2002). Working through family-based problem behavior through activity group therapy. *Clinical Social Work Journal, 30*(4), 419–428.

Trostle, S. (1988). The effects of child-centered group play sessions on social-emotional growth of three- to six-year-old bilingual Puerto Rican children. *Journal of Research in Childhood Education, 3,* 93–106.

Tyndall-Lind, A., Landreth, G., & Giordano, M. (2001). Intensive group play therapy with child witnesses of domestic violence. *International Journal of Play Therapy, 10,* 53–83.

UNICEF (2007). Child protection from violence, exploitation, abuse: Children in conflict and emergencies. Available at www.unicef.org/protection/index_armedconflict.html

U.S. Census Bureau (2012). Table 10. *Resident Population by Race, Hispanic Origin, and Age: 2000 to 2009.* Available at www.census.gov/compendia/statab/2012/tables/12s0010.pdf

U.S. Department of Health and Human Services (2004). *Mental health response to mass violence and terrorism: A training manual.* DHHS Pub. No. SMA 3959. Rockville, MD: Center for Mental Health Services, Substance Abuse and Mental Health Services Administration.

U.S. Department of Health and Human Services (2012). *Foster care FY2003-FY2011 Entries, exits, and numbers of children in care on the last day of each federal fiscal year.* Washington, DC: U.S. Department of Health and Human Services.

Van der Kolk, B.A. (2001). The assessment and treatment of complex PTSD. In R. Yehuda (Ed.), *Traumatic Stress.* Washington, DC: American Psychiatric Press.

Van der Kolk, B.A. (2006). Clinical implications of neuroscience research in PTSD. In R. Yehuda (Ed.), *Psychobiology of posttraumatic stress disorders: A decade of progress* (Vol. 1071, pp. 277–293). Malden, MA: Blackwell.

Van der Kolk, B.A. (2007). The developmental impact of childhood trauma. In L.J. Kirmayer, R. Lemelson, & M. Barad (Eds.), *Understanding trauma: Integrating biological, clinical, and cultural perspectives* (pp. 224–241). New York: Cambridge University Press.

Vander, A.H. (1946). Levels and applications of group therapy: round table. *American Journal of Orthopsychiatry, XIV,* 1944, pp. 478–608. *Psychoanalytic Quarterly, 15,* 552–553.

Van Velsor, P. (2004). Training for successful group work with children: What and how to teach. *Journal for Specialists in Group Work, 29*(1), 137–146.

Wadeson, H. (2010). *Art psychotherapy* (2nd ed.). Hoboken, NJ: John Wiley & Sons.

Wainscott, M.C. (2006). The relationship of depression in middle school adolescents and their school extracurricular activities: A perspective for family therapy. *Dissertation Abstracts International, 66.*

Wakenshaw, M. (2002). *Caring for your grieving child: Engaging activities for dealing with loss and transition.* Oakland, CA: New Harbinger.

Webb, N.B. (2007). *Play therapy with children in crisis: Individual, group, and family treatment* (3rd ed.). New York: Guilford Press.

Weinrib, E. (1983). *Images of self: The sandplay therapy process.* Boston, MA: Sigo Press.

Wells, H.G. (1911). *Floor games.* New York: Arno Press. (Originally published in England. First US edition, 1912, Boston, MA.)

Willis, C.A. (2002). The grieving process in children: Strategies for understanding, educating, and reconciling children's perceptions of death. *Early Childhood Education Journal, 29*(4), 221–226.

Winnicott, D.W. (1989). The squiggle game. In C. Winnicott, R. Shepherd, & M. David (Eds.), *Psychoanalytic explorations* (pp. 299–317). Cambridge, MA: Harvard University Press.

Woltmann, A. (1940). The use of puppets in understanding children. *Mental Hygiene, 24,* 445–458.

Woltmann, A. (1972). Puppetry as a tool in child psychotherapy. *International Journal of Child Psychotherapy, 1,* 84–96.

World Health Organization (WHO). (2003). *Mental health in emergencies.* Geneva: WHO. Retrieved from www5.who.int/mental_health

Yalom, I.D. (1989). *Love's executioner: And other tales of psychotherapy.* New York: Basic Books.

Yalom, I. (2005). *The theory and practice of group psychotherapy* (5th ed.). New York: Basic Books.

Yontef, G., & Jacobs, L. (2005). Gestalt therapy. In R. Corsini & D. Wedding (Eds.), *Current psychotherapies* (7th ed., pp. 299–336). Belmont, CA: Brooks/Cole.

Zalaquett, C., Foley, P., Tillotson, K., Dinsmore, J., & Hof, D. (2008). Multicultural and social justice training for counselor education programs and Colleges of Education: Rewards and challenges. *Journal of Counseling and Development, 86*(3), 323–329.

Index

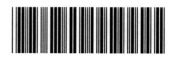